Clinical Utility of ^{18}F NaF PET/CT in Benign and Malignant Disorders

Guest Editor

MOHSEN BEHESHTI, MD

PET CLINICS

www.pet.theclinics.com

Consulting Editor

ABASS ALAVI, MD, PhD (Hon), DSc (Hon)

July 2012 • Volume 7 • Number 3

SAUNDERS an imprint of ELSEVIER, Inc.

W.B. SAUNDERS COMPANY
A Division of Elsevier Inc.

1600 John F. Kennedy Boulevard ● Suite 1800 ● Philadelphia, Pennsylvania 19103-2899

http://www.theclinics.com

PET CLINICS Volume 7, Number 3
July 2012 ISSN 1556-8598, ISBN-13: 978-1-4557-4886-0

Editor: Sarah Barth

PET Clinics (ISSN 1556-8598) is published quarterly by Elsevier Inc., 360 Park Avenue South, New York, NY 10010-1710. Months of issue are January, April, July, and October. Periodicals postage paid at New York, NY, and additional mailing offices. Subscription prices per year are $215.00 (US individuals), $297.00 (US institutions), $110.00 (US students), $244.00 (Canadian individuals), $332.00 (Canadian institutions), $124.00 (Canadian students), $260.00 (foreign individuals), $332.00 (foreign institutions), and $134.00 (foreign students). To receive student and resident rate, orders must be accompanied by name of affiliated institution, date of term, and the signature of program/residency coordinator on institution letterhead. Orders will be billed at individual rate until proof of status is received. Foreign air speed delivery is included in all Clinics subscription prices. All prices are subject to change without notice. POSTMASTER: Send address changes to PET Clinics, Elsevier Health Sciences Division, Subscription Customer Service, 3251 Riverport Lane, Maryland Heights, MO 63043. **Customer Service: 1-800-654-2452 (U.S. and Canada); 314-447-8871 (outside U.S. and Canada). Fax: 314-447-8029. E-mail: journalscustomerservice-usa@elsevier.com (for print support); journalsonlinesupport-usa@elsevier.com (for online support).**

Reprints. For copies of 100 or more of articles in this publication, please contact the Commercial Reprints Department, Elsevier Inc., 360 Park Avenue South, New York, NY 10010-1710. Tel.: 212-633-3812; Fax: 212-462-1935; E-mail: reprints@elsevier.com.

Printed and bound by CPI Group (UK) Ltd, Croydon, CR0 4YY

Transferred to Digital Print 2012

Contributors

CONSULTING EDITOR

ABASS ALAVI, MD, PhD (Hon), DSc (Hon)
Professor of Radiology, Division of Nuclear
Medicine, University of Pennsylvania School of
Medicine, Philadelphia, Pennsylvania

GUEST EDITOR

MOHSEN BEHESHTI, MD, FASNC, FEBNM
Associate Professor in Nuclear Medicine,
Senior Attending Physician, PET-CT Center
LINZ, Nuclear Medicine and Endocrinology,
St. Vincent's Hospital, Linz, Austria

AUTHORS

GAD ABIKHZER, MDCM, FRCPC, ABNM
Department of Nuclear Medicine, Rambam
Health Care Campus, Haifa, Israel

ABASS ALAVI, MD, PhD (Hon), DSc (Hon)
Professor of Radiology, Division of Nuclear
Medicine, University of Pennsylvania School
of Medicine, Philadelphia, Pennsylvania

**SANDIP BASU, MBBS (Hons), DRM, DNB,
MNAMS**
Radiation Medicine Centre, Bhabha Atomic
Research Centre, Tata Memorial Hospital
Annexe, Parel, Mumbai, Maharashtra, India

MOHSEN BEHESHTI, MD FASNC, FEBNM
Associate Professor in Nuclear Medicine,
Senior Attending Physician, PET-CT Center
LINZ, Nuclear Medicine and Endocrinology,
St. Vincent's Hospital, Linz, Austria

GLEN M. BLAKE, PhD
Professor, Osteoporosis Unit, King's College
London, King's Health Partners, Guy's
Hospital, London, United Kingdom

LAURA A. DRUBACH, MD
Assistant Professor in Radiology, Children's
Hospital Boston, Boston, Massachusetts

IGNAC FOGELMAN, MD
Professor, Department of Nuclear Medicine,
King's College London, King's Health Partners,
Guy's Hospital, London, United Kingdom

MICHELLE L. FROST, PhD
Osteoporosis Unit, King's College London,
King's Health Partners, Guy's Hospital,
London, United Kingdom

ANDREI IAGARU, MD
Assistant Professor of Radiology, Division of
Nuclear Medicine, Stanford University Medical
Center, Stanford, California

ORA ISRAEL, MD
Department of Nuclear Medicine, Rambam
Health Care Campus; Ruth and Bruce
Rapaport Faculty of Medicine, Technion–Israel
Institute of Technology, Haifa, Israel

JOHN KENNEDY, PhD
Department of Nuclear Medicine, Rambam
Health Care Campus, Haifa, Israel

WERNER LANGSTEGER, MD, FACE
Department of Nuclear Medicine and
Endocrinology, PET/CT Center LINZ, St
Vincent's Hospital, Linz, Seilerstaette, Austria

AMELIA E. B. MOORE, PhD
Osteoporosis Unit, King's College London,
King's Health Partners, Guy's Hospital,
London, United Kingdom

CAMILA MOSCI, MD
Post-Doctoral Fellow, Division of Nuclear
Medicine, Stanford University Medical Center,
Stanford, California

MUSIB SIDDIQUE, PhD
Osteoporosis Unit, King's College London,
King's Health Partners, Guy's Hospital,
London, United Kingdom

KLAUS STROBEL, MD
Department of Radiology and Nuclear
Medicine, Cantonal Hospital Lucerne, Lucerne,
Switzerland

REZA VALI, MD, FEBNM
Department of Radiology and Nuclear
Medicine, Hospital for Sick Children, Toronto,
Ontario, Canada

Contents

Nuclear physicians in many centers nowadays have the choice of using different nuclear bone-imaging modalities. ^{18}F-labeled sodium fluoride (NaF) PET with computed tomography (PET/CT) is a promising tool for the evaluation of benign bone disease. The indications for NaF PET/CT in clinical practice are probably the same as those established for ^{99m}Tc-labeled methylene diphosphonate bone scintigraphy and single-photon emission computed tomography (SPECT)/CT. At present only preliminary data, often with a limited number of patients and lacking comparison with ^{99m}Tc-MDP SPECT/CT, are available. This article reviews the available literature and summarizes the authors' experience with NaF PET/CT in benign bone disease.

Diagnostic imaging plays a major role in the evaluation of patients with malignant bone disease. ^{18}F-Labeled sodium fluoride (^{18}F NaF) is a positron-emitting radiopharmaceutical with desirable characteristics (rapid blood clearance and bone uptake) for high-quality functional imaging of the skeleton. In addition to higher sensitivity and specificity, ^{18}F NaF PET combined with computed tomography (PET/CT) allows for shorter imaging time, thus improving patients' convenience and benefiting the overall workflow of the imaging facility. Although as yet no robust evidence-based data exist, this article summarizes the published data currently available on the role of ^{18}F NaF PET/CT in the assessment of malignant bone disease.

Studies of bone remodeling using bone biopsy and biochemical markers of bone turnover measured in serum and urine are important for investigating how new treatments for osteoporosis affect bone metabolism. Positron emission tomography with ^{18}F sodium fluoride (^{18}F NaF PET) for studying bone metabolism complements these conventional methods. Unlike biochemical markers, which measure the integrated response to treatment across the whole skeleton, ^{18}F NaF PET can distinguish changes occurring at sites of clinically important osteoporotic fractures. Future studies using ^{18}F NaF PET may illuminate current clinical problems, such as the possible association between long-term treatment with bisphosphonates and atypical fractures of the femur.

Skeletal imaging of children with fluorine-18 (^{18}F) NaF harnesses the superior imaging characteristics of positron emission tomography (PET) and the improved biodistribution of the fluoride tracer compared with standard nuclear techniques, resulting in excellent quality images. Bone malignancy in children is less common than in adults, and the evaluation of benign skeletal disorders represents a larger fraction of indications in the pediatric versus adult population. [18]F NaF PET imaging has been successfully applied to various benign disorders, particularly trauma and sports medicine applications.

The skeletal system is the third most common site of metastases after the lungs and liver, and 80% of all reported metastatic bone disease is in patients with breast and prostate cancer. At present there are an unprecedented number of novel molecular imaging agents potentially available for the assessment of bone metastases in different cancer. This review assesses the role of PET in the imaging of skeletal metastases, focusing on the specific PET tracers (fluorodeoxyglucose, choline derivatives, and so forth), in comparison with [18]F NaF as a nonspecific bone-seeking PET agent.

Conventional planar and SPECT bone scintigraphy has long been used and familiarity with this tracer and imaging technique is excellent. [18]F NaF PET/CT represents an alternative tracer and imaging modality for the assessment of the skeleton, with the potential to become the gold standard in functional bone imaging. This article compares the pharmacokinetics, protocols, clinical performance, and cost-effectiveness of the 2 modalities. Technological advances and future directions of both modalities are also discussed.

Detection of early ongoing cardiovascular molecular calcification and its quantification through ^{18}F-labeled sodium fluoride ([18]F NaF) PET/computed tomography (CT) imaging has been a recent addition to the diagnostic armamentarium of molecular imaging for the atherosclerotic process. At present, visual detection of molecular calcification as well as its regional quantification on ([18]F NaF) PET/CT are suboptimal, mainly because of the very low degree of uptake of this radiotracer in the heart and major vessels, and hence subject to the partial volume effect. Calculation of cardiovascular [18]F NaF uptake in the heart and arterial wall using automated software is an innovative approach.

PET Clinics

GOAL STATEMENT

The goal of the *PET Clinics* is to keep practicing radiologists and radiology residents up to date with current clinical practice in positron emission tomography by providing timely articles reviewing the state of the art in patient care.

ACCREDITATION

PET Clinics is planned and implemented in accordance with the Essential Areas and Policies of the Accreditation Council for Continuing Medical Education (ACCME) through the joint sponsorship of the University of Virginia School of Medicine and Elsevier. The University of Virginia School of Medicine is accredited by the ACCME to provide continuing medical education for physicians.

The University of Virginia School of Medicine designates this enduring material activity for a maximum of 15 *AMA PRA Category 1 Credit(s)™ for each issue,* 60 credits per year. Physicians should only claim credit commensurate with the extent of their participation in the activity.

The American Medical Association has determined that physicians not licensed in the US who participate in this CME enduring material activity are eligible for a maximum of 15 *AMA PRA Category 1 Credit(s)™* for each issue, 60 credits per year.

Credit can be earned by reading the text material, taking the CME examination online at http://www.theclinics.com/home/cme, and completing the evaluation. After taking the test, you will be required to review any and all incorrect answers. Following completion of the test and evaluation, your credit will be awarded and you may print your certificate.

FACULTY DISCLOSURE/CONFLICT OF INTEREST

The University of Virginia School of Medicine, as an ACCME accredited provider, endorses and strives to comply with the Accreditation Council for Continuing Medical Education (ACCME) Standards of Commercial Support, Commonwealth of Virginia statutes, University of Virginia policies and procedures, and associated federal and private regulations and guidelines on the need for disclosure and monitoring of proprietary and financial interests that may affect the scientific integrity and balance of content delivered in continuing medical education activities under our auspices.

The University of Virginia School of Medicine requires that all CME activities accredited through this institution be developed independently and be scientifically rigorous, balanced and objective in the presentation/discussion of its content, theories and practices.

All authors/editors participating in an accredited CME activity are expected to disclose to the readers relevant financial relationships with commercial entities occurring within the past 12 months (such as grants or research support, employee, consultant, stock holder, member of speakers bureau, etc.). The University of Virginia School of Medicine will employ appropriate mechanisms to resolve potential conflicts of interest to maintain the standards of fair and balanced education to the reader. Questions about specific strategies can be directed to the Office of Continuing Medical Education, University of Virginia School of Medicine, Charlottesville, Virginia.

The faculty and staff of the University of Virginia Office of Continuing Medical Education have no financial affiliations to disclose.

The authors/editors listed below have identified no professional or financial affiliations for themselves or their spouse/ partner:
Gad Abikhzer, MDCM, FRCPC, ABNM; Abass Alavi, MD, PhD (Hon), DSc (Hon) (Consulting Editor); Sarah Barth, (Acquisitions Editor); Sandip Basu, MBBS (Hons), DRM, DNB, MNAMS; Moshen Beheshti, MD, FASNC, FEBNM (Guest Editor); Laura A. Drubach, MD; Ignac Fogelman, MD; John Kennedy, PhD; Werner Langsteger, MD, FACE; Camila Mosci, MD; Patrice Rehm, MD (Test Editor); Musib Siddique, PhD; Klaus Strobel, MD; Reza Vali, MD, FEBNM.

The authors/editors listed below identified the following professional or financial affiliations for themselves or their spouse/partner:
Glen M. Blake, PhD receives research support from Novartis.
Michelle L. Frost, PhD receives research support from Novartis Pharma.
Andrei Iagaru, MD is on the Advisory Board for Siemens Molecular Imaging.
Ora Israel, MD is on the Advisory Committee for General Electric Healthcare, and receives research support from UltraSPECT.
Amelia E.B. Moore, PhD receives research support from King's College London.

Disclosure of Discussion of Non-FDA Approved Uses for Pharmaceutical Products and/or Medical Devices
The University of Virginia School of Medicine, as an ACCME provider, requires that all faculty presenters identify and disclose any off-label uses for pharmaceutical and medical device products. The University of Virginia School of Medicine recommends that each physician fully review all the available data on new products or procedures prior to clinical use.

TO ENROLL
To enroll in the PET Clinics Continuing Medical Education program, call customer service at 1-800-654-2452 or visit us online at www.theclinics.com/home/cme. The CME program is available to subscribers for an additional fee of $196.00.

Preface

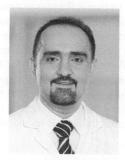

Mohsen Beheshti, MD, FEBNM
Guest Editor

Bone imaging using ^{18}F-labeled sodium fluoride (^{18}F NaF) was first described in 1962; nevertheless, the clinical relevance of this method has only started to be appreciated recently. The co-appearance with gamma camera introduction and Tc-99m-labeled diphosphonates application, as well as insufficient positron emission tomography (PET) data acquisition technology, were the most important reasons for the lack of ^{18}F NaF PET application in the clinical routine practise.

With the improvements of new PET scanners, high-resolution imaging of bone became a reality; hence, ^{18}F NaF was reintroduced for clinical and research investigations.

In this issue of *PET Clinics*, we have focused on the clinical utility of ^{18}F NaF PET and hybrid PET/computed tomography (CT) in benign and malignant disorders.

An overview of the role of ^{18}F NaF PET in the assessment of benign bone imaging is presented in the first article. Despite limited data in this concern, Drs Strobel and Vali discuss the role of ^{18}F NaF PET in the assessment of metabolic, inflammatory, and traumatic bone disease, benign tumors, as well as grafts and bone vitality. In the second article, Dr Iagaru and colleagues from Stanford University Medical Center describe the value of ^{18}F NaF PET in primary as well as metastatic bone disease focusing on the breast, lung, and prostate cancers as the most common cancers that metastasize to the skeletal system. This article, in combination with the fifth article from our group in PET-CT Center Linz, St. Vincent's Hospital, Austria, explores the role of PET imaging using specific radiotracers in investigating

skeletal involvement by cancers. The authors focus on the significance and implications of the osseous abnormalities visualized by PET imaging using specific PET tracers (eg, fluorodeoxyglucose, choline derivatives, etc) as opposed to those seen by either morphological imaging (eg, CT) or nonspecific functional imaging modalities such as bone scintigraphy and ^{18}F NaF PET.

The dynamic, changing, and progressive pattern of abnormality associated with bone metastases, beginning with bone marrow involvement (without morphological changes), then generally osteoblastic but sometimes osteoclastic changes (positive functional and morphological findings), and finally progressing to densely sclerotic lesions without any metabolic activity, is explained in these articles. The authors conclude that specific PET tracers are promising in the early detection of bone metastases, when it is still confined to the bone marrow, which is most desirable for accurate assessment of disease. The impact of PET imaging using specific PET tracers as well as ^{18}F NaF, as a nonspecific bone seeking PET agent, is also reviewed in these articles.

In the third article, Drs Blake, Fogelman, and their group at King's College, London, describe the quantitative ^{18}F NaF PET imaging and its role in the assessment of metabolic bone imaging and their response to the therapy monitoring. They showed that ^{18}F NaF PET provides a novel tool for studying bone metabolism that can measure the effects of treatment at specific sites such as the spine and hip. Clinical pediatric indications of ^{18}F NaF PET/CT is summarized in the next article by Dr Drubach from Children's Hospital, Boston.

PET Clin 7 (2012) ix–x
doi:10.1016/j.cpet.2012.04.008

In the sixth article, Dr Israel and her colleagues from Rambam Health Care Campus in Israel deal with important issues concerning the potentials of ^{18}F NaF PET comparing conventional bone scanning and analyze tracer characteristics, performance indices, and cost effectiveness of each modality.

In the final article, the value of ^{18}F NaF PET in the detection and global quantification of cardiovascular molecular calcification as part of the atherosclerotic process is discussed. Professor Alavi from University of Pennsylvania and his colleagues discuss a novel approach for assessing global molecular calcification, particularly in subclinical atherosclerosis, and raise the importance of ^{18}F NaF PET in depicting ongoing active molecular calcification in the atherosclerotic plaques, which theoretically could be before the heralding of structural calcification detectable by CT.

In this issue of *PET Clinics*, we portray the utility of ^{18}F NaF PET in a variety of clinical settings and

hope that this issue provides useful information to all interested readers.

I take this opportunity to thank Professor Abass Alavi for all his contributions in the field of molecular imaging and in particular for inviting me to contribute in this issue of *PET Clinics*. I would like to thank Professor Werner Langsteger for his support in providing an international list of expert contributors. I also thank Sarah Barth for her excellent coordination from initial concept to the final publication. I dedicate this work to my wife and my two sons.

Mohsen Beheshti, MD, FEBNM
Department of Nuclear Medicine and
Endocrinology, PET/CT Center LINZ
St Vincent's Hospital, Seilerstaette 4
A-4020, Linz, Austria

E-mail address:
mohsen.beheshti@bhs.at

^{18}F NaF PET/CT Versus Conventional Bone Scanning in the Assessment of Benign Bone Disease

Klaus Strobel, MD[a],*, Reza Vali, MD, FEBNM[b]

KEYWORDS

- ^{18}F NaF PET/CT • Benign bone disease • Bone tumor • Trauma • Bone graft • Joint prosthesis

KEY POINTS

- ^{18}F-labeled sodium fluoride (^{18}F NaF) PET with computed tomography (PET/CT) is a very promising tool for the evaluation of benign bone disease.
- Insufficiency fracture, occult fractures, osteoarthritis, osteoid osteoma, failed back surgery, or child abuse are auspicious indications of fluoride PET/CT.
- With development in PET technology and more availability of PET/CT machines and routine performance of dynamic quantitative imaging, ^{18}F NaF PET/CT will probably play a major role in the assessment of various benign bone diseases in the near future.
- Further comparative studies are needed with larger patient populations and direct comparison of ^{18}F NaF PET/CT with established imaging modalities such as technetium-based bone scanning and SPECT/CT.

INTRODUCTION

^{18}F-labeled sodium fluoride (^{18}F NaF) positron emission tomography/computed tomography (PET/CT) is a very promising tool for the evaluation of benign bone disease. Conventional bone scanning has traditionally been used for evaluation of a wide variety of abnormalities. Since the availability of ^{99}Tc-labeled bone-seeking tracers has improved again after some months of supply crisis, and with the increasing installation of new-generation single-photon emission computed tomography/computed tomography (SPECT/CT) devices, nuclear physicians in many large centers have the choice of using different nuclear bone-imaging modalities.[1] The indications for ^{18}F NaF PET/CT in clinical practice are probably the same as those established for ^{99m}Tc-labeled diphosphonate (eg, methylene diphosphonate [MDP]) conventional bone scintigraphy (BS) and SPECT/CT. However, comparative studies are still needed for benign bone diseases. Such studies have been performed successfully for bone metastases.[2] At present only preliminary data, often with a limited number of patients and lacking comparison with ^{99m}Tc-MDP SPECT/CT, are available. This article reviews the available literature and summarizes the authors' experience with ^{18}F NaF PET/CT in benign bone disease.

METABOLIC BONE DISEASE

^{18}F NaF PET/CT has been used in different metabolic bone diseases. In the authors' experience, ^{18}F NaF PET/CT can be very helpful for the

[a] Department of Radiology and Nuclear Medicine, Cantonal Hospital Lucerne, Spitalstrasse, 6000 Lucerne 16, Switzerland; [b] Department of Radiology and Nuclear Medicine, Hospital for Sick Children, 555 University Avenue, Toronto, ON M5G 1X8, Canada
* Corresponding author. Luzerner Kantonsspital, 6000 Luzern 16, Switzerland.
E-mail address: klaus.strobel@luks.ch

PET Clin 7 (2012) 249–261
doi:10.1016/j.cpet.2012.04.007
1556-8598/12/$ – see front matter © 2012 Elsevier Inc. All rights reserved.

evaluation of bone involvement in hyperparathyroidism. It is a very sensitive method for detecting the areas of increased bone turnover or insufficiency fractures. Moreover, the CT part is useful for the evaluation of the extension of brown tumors and for assessment of bone stability (**Fig. 1**).

Some investigators have used ^{18}F NaF PET/CT in research settings to measure bone turnover noninvasively, and have found a good correlation with histomorphometry.[3] Messa and colleagues[4] described a good correlation between ^{18}F NaF metabolism and levels of serum markers such as alkaline phosphatase and parathyroid hormone in

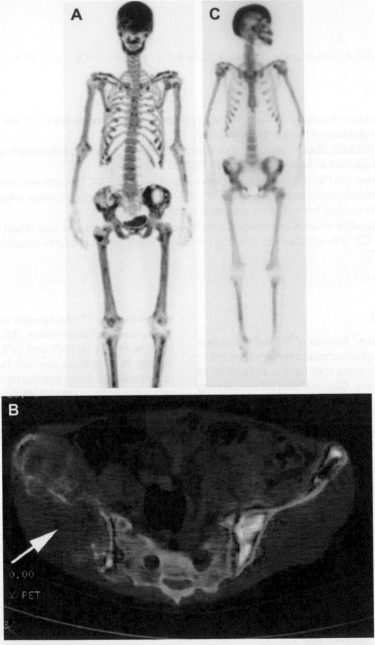

Fig. 1. A patient with severe hyperparathyroidism. ^{18}F NaF PET/CT maximum-intensity projection (MIP) image (*A*) shows increased bone turnover (superscan) in the whole skeleton with some "cold" areas, for example in the pelvis. On the axial fused image (*B*), a large brown tumor (*arrow*) is visible. (*C*) Corresponding conventional bone superscan of the same patient.

patients with renal osteodystrophy. [18]F NaF PET study was useful in differentiating low-turnover from high-turnover lesions of renal osteodystrophy, and provided quantitative estimates of osseous cell activity.

[18]F NaF PET/CT was successfully used to investigate bone metabolism in osteoporosis. Uchida and colleagues[5] measured the effects of bisphosphonate treatment on bone metabolism with [18]F NaF PET/CT. [18]F NaF PET/CT can be used to detect insufficiency fractures in patients with osteoporosis because of its high sensitivity.

INFLAMMATORY/RHEUMATOLOGIC BONE DISEASE

Rheumatologic disease involving the bones and joints, such as rheumatoid arthritis and spondyloarthropathies, are classic indications for conventional BS. The distribution pattern of involved joints, the intensity of uptake, and the positivity of the early-phase images are useful for the detection, characterization, and staging of various inflammatory diseases, and help to guide the treatment.

Despite the established value of BS in inflammatory diseases, there are important limitations. Several publications have shown that BS is not sensitive enough to detect sacroiliitis. In a systematic literature review, it was positive only in 52% of the patients with established ankylosing spondylitis (AS) and in 49.4% of the patients with probable sacroiliitis.[6] This low sensitivity might be one of the reasons why in many institutions magnetic resonance (MR) imaging replaced BS as the first-line imaging tool in patients with suspected AS or other spondyloarthropathies. MR imaging is more sensitive and has superior performance to BS in detecting sacroiliitis in the early stage.[7,8]

Experience with [18]F NaF PET/CT in patients with rheumatologic disease is limited. Strobel and colleagues[9] compared the performance of [18]F NaF PET/CT and BS regarding the detection of sacroiliitis. The study included 15 patients with AS fulfilling the modified New York criteria; 13 patients with mechanical back pain served as the control group. The investigators implemented a ratio between uptake in the sacroiliac joints (SIJ) and the sacrum (S) similar to the measurement that was established for BS. Using a SIJ/S ratio of greater than 1.3 as the threshold for sacroiliitis, [18]F NaF PET/CT was significantly superior to BS, with a sensitivity of 80% in per-patient analysis (BS: 47%). Another advantage of [18]F NaF PET/CT imaging is the possibility to obtain morphologic information about the joints with CT (Fig. 2). Because the scintigraphic activity of the involved joint decreases in patients with advanced ankylosis of the SIJ, the morphologic information of the low-dose CT part of the study usually leads to the correct diagnosis in such cases.

Patients with spondyloarthropathies may also suffer from enthesiopathies and arthritis. In the authors' experience, [18]F NaF PET/CT is a very sensitive tool for identifying sites of enthesitis (Fig. 3). Because of the rapid blood clearance and first-pass extraction of [18]F NaF, early-phase images (such as what we are familiar with in conventional bone scans), are difficult to obtain.[10] This fact might be a limitation in patients with arthritis, because the important information of early uptake in the periarticular soft tissue as an indicator for active arthritis might be missed on an [18]F NaF PET scan (Fig. 4). Other investigators showed that early-phase images, 2 minutes after injection, might show increased regional blood flow in the inflammatory or infectious diseases.[11] As already mentioned, MR imaging also plays an evolving role in imaging patients with inflammatory disease. With increasing implementation and velocity of whole-body MR imaging, it becomes a competitor regarding whole-body "staging" of inflammatory diseases.[12] Most of the actual MR imaging protocols include the axial skeleton sparing the peripheral joints. In a preliminary study, Fischer and colleagues[13] compared whole-body MR imaging and [18]F NaF PET/CT in 10 patients with AS. The investigators concluded that increased [18]F NaF uptake on PET correlated only modestly with bone marrow edema on MR imaging in the spine ($\kappa = 0.25$) whereas there was a better correlation in the SIJ ($\kappa = 0.64$). These initial results indicate that bone marrow edema on MR imaging and increased uptake on [18]F NaF PET/CT do not represent the same pathological situation. Nuclear medicine techniques may detect increased bone turnover, not only caused by inflammation but mainly by osteoproliferative reparative changes in the chronic stage of the disease. [18]F NaF PET/CT may also be useful for the evaluation of disease progression and response to therapy in inflammatory diseases. Baraliakos and colleagues[14] showed that treatment with the anti–tumor necrosis factor α antibody infliximab does not completely inhibit, but may decelerate radiographic progression in patients with AS over 4 years. [18]F NaF PET/CT might be an interesting tool for the monitoring of therapy response in this particular patient population.

TRAUMA

Conventional radiography is the first-line imaging modality to detect fractures, especially in the

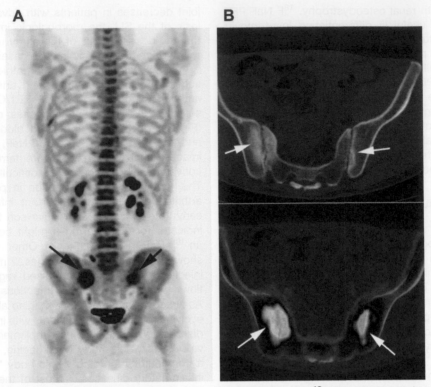

Fig. 2. A young patient with chronic pain in the lumbar spine and pelvis. ^{18}F NaF PET/CT MIP image (*A*) shows markedly increased uptake in both iliosacral joints (*arrows*). On the axial fused image (*B*), additional erosions and sclerotic changes in the iliac bone and sacrum are seen (*arrows*). A diagnosis of ankylosing spondylitis was established.

extremities. Complex fractures involving the joints or occult fractures that are not visible on standard radiographs are usually imaged with CT because of the rapidity and wide availability of CT imaging. The value of ^{18}F NaF PET/CT in trauma has already been discussed in the published studies. The results are promising in child abuse, in which highly sensitive modalities are needed to detect new and old fractures in the whole body skeleton. Drubach and colleagues[15] compared the classic skeletal survey with ^{18}F NaF PET in 22 infants with the suspicion of fractures attributable to child abuse. ^{18}F NaF PET was shown to be more sensitive in general by detecting more lesions compared with radiographs (200 vs 156). ^{18}F NaF PET was especially more sensitive in the detection of thoracic (ribs, sternum, clavicle, scapula) and posterior rib fractures, but inferior regarding the detection of metaphyseal fractures, the typical presentation of child abuse. ^{18}F NaF PET/CT is very sensitive in the detection of all kinds of fractures including occult fractures in complex anatomic regions (**Fig. 5**), insufficiency fractures,[16] and pathologic fractures. At present, literature

regarding this topic is limited to case reports, and the additional value of ^{18}F NaF PET/CT in comparison with the other established imaging methods has not been completely evaluated.

EVALUATION OF JOINT PROSTHESIS

With increasing life expectancy, prosthetic joint replacement surgeries are becoming more frequent. Despite the advances in orthopedic reconstructive and reparative techniques, complications including loosening, infection, dislocation, and fracture still occur in a considerable number of patients. The definitive diagnosis of these complications is essential for optimal patient management. In particular, infection should be differentiated from aseptic loosening, because the clinical presentation and histopathologic changes are similar.

Plain radiography is considered the primary imaging modality for the assessment of patients after hip or knee arthroplasties. However, they are only helpful when some abnormalities such as gross prosthetic malpositions, fractures, or wide radiolucencies are seen. Three-phase conventional

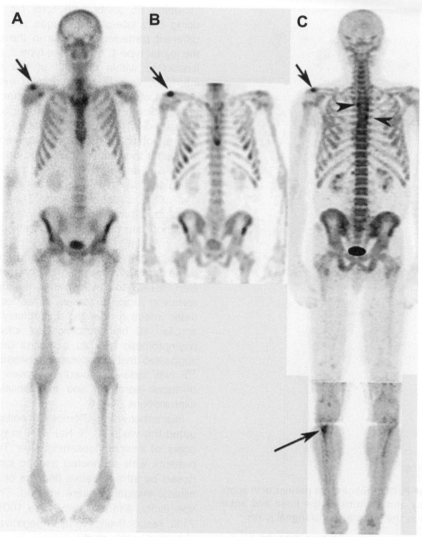

Fig. 3. Comparison of planar conventional bone scintigraphy (*A*), partial body SPECT (*B*), and ^{18}F NaF PET/CT (*C*) in a patient with ankylosing spondylitis. On the planar images and SPECT views, alteration of the right acromiocla-vicular joint is seen (*arrows*). Involvement of multiple costovertebral joints (*arrowheads*) and enthesiopathy at the right tibial tuberosity (*long arrow*) was better detected by the ^{18}F NaF PET/CT.

bone scan is considered one of the initial methods for the assessment of complications after arthro-plasty. The negative predictive value of a 3-phase bone scan for the detection of loosening or infec-tion is very high, making it a good modality for ruling out these complications. However, it suffers from sufficient specificity. Correlative ^{67}Ga imaging, ^{111}In-labeled white blood cells (WBC), 99mTc sulfur colloid marrow studies, and ^{111}In-labeled poly-clonal immunoglobulin G (IgG) scanning have been used to increase the specificity of the 3-phase bone scan.[17] ^{111}In-labeled WBC scan is considered the gold-standard method for the evaluation of infection. However, it has its own limitations. The problems with in vitro labeling process, availability,

and the need for correlative bone marrow imaging make it difficult to be done routinely. Addition of the ^{99m}Tc-MDP SPECT/CT technique to bone scanning was shown to be helpful by providing the anatomic information to the functional bone scan and consequently improving its specificity.[18] However, the CT part may be affected by the arti-facts resulting from the presence of the prosthetic metallic devices.[17] In a study by Hirschmann and colleagues,[19] ^{99m}Tc-MDP SPECT/CT was useful for the diagnosis and guidance of treatment management in patients with painful knees after total knee arthroplasty (TKA), particularly in patients with patellofemoral problems and malpositioned or loose knee endoprosthesis.

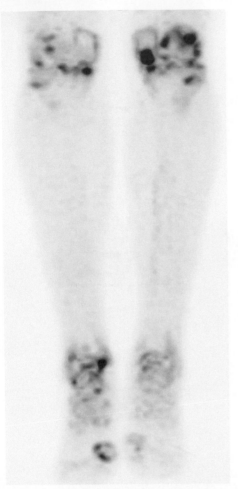

Fig. 4. ^{18}F NaF PET/CT images of a patient with spondylarthropathy and arthritis of the knee and ankle joints as well as the metatarsophalangeal joints.

Initial experience with ^{18}F NaF PET/CT for the evaluation of complications after joint replacements was very promising. Kobayashi and colleagues[20] performed a prospective study including 65 joints with total hip arthroplasty, using only late-phase images and proposing 3 different patterns of uptake in the evaluation of the joints: type 1, no uptake; type 2, minor uptake limited to within one-half of the bone-implant interface, type 3, major uptake extending over one-half of the bone-implant interface. Maximum standardized uptake value (SUV$_{max}$) was also measured at all sites of increased uptake. There was a significant difference between the SUV$_{max}$ values for the aseptic and septic loosening cases. Sensitivity and specificity using pattern type 3 for the diagnosis of infected arthroplasty was 95% and 98%, respectively.[20] The investigators concluded that the proposed uptake pattern classification can be performed relatively easily, and that ^{18}F NaF PET/CT is very promising in the differentiation of loosening and infection. The same group of researchers evaluated the use of ^{18}F NaF PET/CT to determine the appropriate tissue-sampling region in cases of suspected periprosthetic infection after hip arthroplasty.[21] The study enrolled 23 hips suspicious of infection and 23 asymptomatic hips as a control group. Findings suggested that preoperative assessment of major ^{18}F NaF uptake markedly improves the accuracy of tissue sampling and the sensitivity of tissue examinations (**Fig. 6**).

In another study, Sterner and colleagues[22] evaluated the value of ^{18}F NaF PET in the early diagnosis of aseptic loosening after TKA. Fourteen patients with suspected aseptic loosening diagnosed by intraoperative findings or by long-term clinical evaluation were imaged. The sensitivity, specificity, and accuracy were 100%, 56%, and 71%, respectively. No false-negative results were detected in this study.

To the authors' knowledge no studies have been published that compare the accuracy of 3-phase BS and ^{18}F NaF PET/CT in patients after

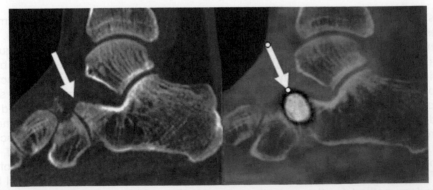

Fig. 5. A patient with unclear foot pain 3 months after trauma and normal conventional radiographs. CT (*left*) and fused ^{18}F NaF PET/CT (*right*) images showed an old fracture of the anterior process of the calcaneus with markedly increased uptake (*arrows*).

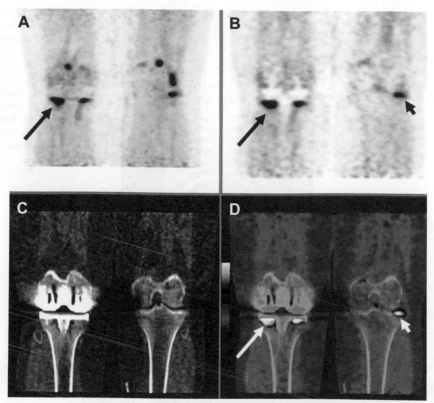

Fig. 6. A patient with knee prosthesis for 6 years. MIP (*A*), coronal [18]F NaF PET (*B*), and fused PET/CT (*C, D*) images show increased uptake at the tibial component interface (*arrows*) suspicious for loosening. On the left side, increased uptake in the lateral femorotibial joint is evident, due to osteoarthritis (*short arrows*).

arthroplasty. Rajender and colleagues[23] presented a comparative study of 3-phase bone scan, [18]F NaF PET/CT, and ^{18}F-fluorodeoxyglucose (FDG) in 46 patients with painful hip prosthesis. The accuracy of bone scan, [18]F NaF PET/CT, and ^{18}F-FDG PET/CT was 84%, 91%, and 94%, respectively. Of note, no significant difference was observed between the SUV_{max} of the loosened arthroplasties and those that were infected. Studies regarding the performance of ^{18}F-FDG PET/CT in the assessment of joint replacement complications are contradictory, reporting accuracies between 67% and 95%.[24–26]

With the new developments in PET technology, more availability of PET/CT machines, and better performance of dynamic quantitative imaging, [18]F NaF PET/CT will probably play a major role in the future; however, at present conventional bone scanning maintains its position in clinical situations requiring a 3-phase bone study.[27]

BENIGN BONE TUMORS

Studies regarding the evaluation of benign bone tumors with [18]F NaF PET/CT are limited. In the authors' experience, [18]F NaF PET/CT can serve

as an alternative to ^{99m}Tc-MDP SPECT/CT for some interesting indications such as the identification of osteoid osteoma in complex anatomic regions like the axial skeleton or the wrists and feet (**Fig. 7**). MR imaging might be misleading in the detection of osteoid osteoma. The combination of increased scintigraphic focal uptake and corresponding nidus in the CT part of the [18]F NaF PET/CT or ^{99m}Tc-MDP SPECT/CT study usually lead to the correct diagnosis of this important and effectively treatable lesion.[28–30] Because of the relatively high uptake in some incidentally detectable benign bone lesions such as enchondroma, [18]F NaF PET may lead to overdiagnosis. Careful analysis and correlation with the CT part is mandatory to avoid misinterpretation.

ASSESSMENT OF GRAFTS AND BONE VIABILITY
Osteonecrosis Jaw

As initial studies demonstrated the value of ^{99m}Tc-MDP SPECT/CT for the assessment of chronic osteomyelitis and osteonecrosis of the jaw, a first study by Wilde and colleagues[31] addressed the performance of [18]F NaF PET/CT regarding this disease. The investigators compared [18]F NaF

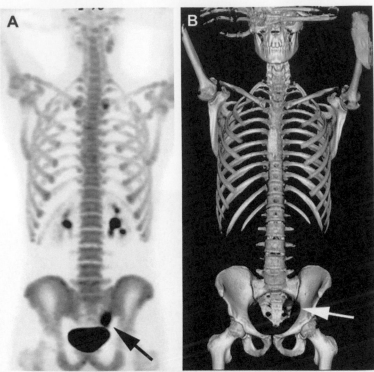

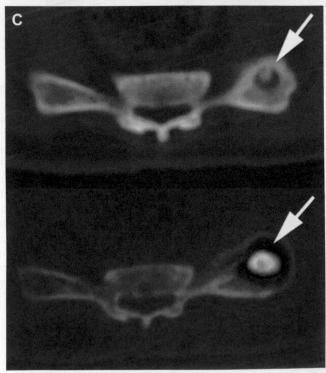

Fig. 7. A young patient with pain in the pelvis. ¹⁸F NaF MIP image (*A*), fused 3-dimensional (3D) image (*B*), and axial fused PET/CT image (*C*) showed focally increased uptake (*arrows*) in the sacrum corresponding to a lesion with a typical nidus in the CT (*upper panel, C*). Diagnosis of an osteoid osteoma was established and was confirmed histologically after resection.

PET/CT and ¹⁸F-FDG PET/CT in 9 patients with bisphosphonate-related osteonecrosis of the jaw. Uptake of the ¹⁸F NaF significantly exceeded the ¹⁸F-FDG activity, making it a very sensitive tool to detect osteonecrosis of the jaw. Comparative studies between ⁹⁹ᵐTc-MDP SPECT/CT and ¹⁸F-FDG PET regarding therapy response assessment in treated osteonecrosis of the jaw indicate a superiority of the ^{18}F-FDG, because bone-seeking agents often lag behind the clinical improvement.[32]

Hip Osteonecrosis

In daily clinical routine, conventional radiographs followed by MR imaging are the first-line imaging modalities in patients with the suspicion for osteonecrosis of the femoral head. Dasa and colleagues[33] investigated the additional value of ^{18}F NaF PET/CT in 17 hips of 11 patients with osteonecrosis of the femoral head compared with MR imaging and SPECT. In 9 hips, additional foci of uptake in the acetabulum were found that were not seen on MR imaging and SPECT. Although the importance of this finding remains unproven, the investigators suggested that acetabular uptake might indicate a prognostic relevant finding regarding progression of the disease.

Bone Grafts

Once conventional BS was established as a method to assess bone graft healing and viability, studies started to evaluate the performance of ^{18}F NaF PET/CT. Brenner and colleagues[34] performed dynamic ^{18}F NaF PET studies in 34 patients for the evaluation of cancellous and full bone grafts of the limbs, and concluded that ^{18}F NaF PET is a promising tool to assess normal healing of bone grafts. Other investigators showed the same results with ^{18}F NaF PET/CT in the assessment of bone graft healing at other sites, including allogenic hip arthroplasty and grafts in maxillofacial surgery.[35,36]

^{18}F NaF PET/CT has been used to study incorporation of anterior cruciate ligament grafts. Secure incorporation of the graft in the bony tunnel is crucial for stable ligament function. Sörensen and colleagues[37] performed sequential ^{18}F NaF PET/CT scans 1 day, 3 weeks, and 7 months or 22 months after surgery in 8 young patients. The highest ^{18}F NaF uptake was found 3 weeks after surgery, with persistent increased activity after 7 months and near normalization after 22 months. The investigators concluded that complete incorporation lasts longer than previously expected, with important impact on postoperative rehabilitation.

Degenerative Diseases

Degenerative diseases are accompanied by increased bone metabolism, making ^{18}F NaF PET/CT a sensitive tool for the detection of osteoarthritic lesions in the skeleton. It is especially useful in complex anatomic structures with multiple small joints, bones, and ligaments such as the foot, in which evaluation with planar bone scans or radiographs might be limited. Fischer and colleagues[38] evaluated the performance of ^{18}F NaF PET/CT in 28 patients with unclear foot pain (**Fig. 8**). Most of these patients underwent CT or MR imaging previously, with inconclusive results. The additive value of ^{18}F NaF PET/CT on therapeutic management was investigated. A variety of abnormalities such as osteoarthritis, painful accessory bones (os trigonum, os tibiale externum), or inflammatory lesions (plantar fasciitis and subtalar osteoarthritis) were found. In 46% of the patients the therapeutic management was changed as a result of the ^{18}F NaF PET/CT findings.

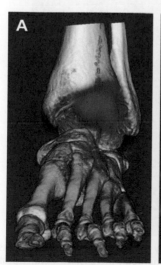 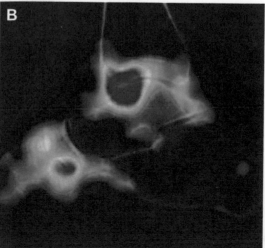

Fig. 8. 3D fused ^{18}F NaF PET/CT image (A) and sagittal fused image (B) of a patient with multiple sites of osteoarthritis in the foot involving the upper ankle, lower ankle, and chopart joints.

In the authors' experience ^{18}F NaF PET/CT, not surprisingly, delivers results comparable with those of conventional BS with ^{99m}Tc-MDP SPECT/CT regarding abnormalities in the foot,[39] but no comparative studies are available thus far. Because of the high ^{18}F NaF uptake in all sites of bone alterations, this method can lead to overdiagnosis. Samarin and colleagues[40] observed sites of increased ^{18}F NaF uptake in 23 of 32 asymptomatic feet, and only 2 of these patients developed pain related to the ^{18}F NaF uptake in the follow-up period. Significantly higher ^{18}F NaF uptake was observed in the symptomatic feet compared with the asymptomatic ones, and it was concluded that low-grade ^{18}F NaF uptake is common in asymptomatic feet and that the intensity of uptake may help to identify the clinically relevant lesions.

MISCELLANEOUS INDICATIONS
Back Pain and Failed Back Surgery

Back pain is a frequent symptom that is often difficult to treat. Initial experience with ^{18}F NaF PET/CT was promising. Ovadia and colleagues[41] found a high rate of positive ^{18}F NaF PET/CT scans in 15 adolescent patients with unclear back pain and inconclusive conventional imaging. The predominant pathological features included spondylolysis, fractures, and osteoid osteoma. A comparison with ^{99m}Tc-MDP SPECT/CT was not directly performed in this population. Another group investigated the relatively high number of 94 young patients with back pain and found the potential source of pain in 55%.[42]

Another interesting field for ^{18}F NaF PET/CT is failed back surgery. There are many reasons for a persistent or recurrent pain after spinal surgery with fusion operations. Metal loosening or fracture, nonunion or pseudarthrosis, suprafusional or infrafusional degeneration, insufficiency fractures, and infection are some of the possible complications. In the authors' experience, the combination of a morphologic assessment of the metal and bone together with the metabolic information of increased bone turnover can identify complications in many cases (Fig. 9). Cervical and lumbar intercorporeal fusions are sometimes performed to treat symptomatic segmental degeneration or instability in the cervical and lumbar spine.

The incorporation of cages after intercorporeal fusion surgery can be evaluated with ^{18}F NaF PET/CT. Fischer and colleagues[43] imaged 30 cages in 20 patients with a wide range of 2 to 116 months' follow-up after the fusion surgery. Forty-eight percent of the cages with a time interval of more than 1 year after surgery showed increased

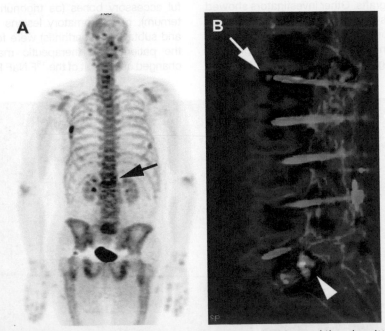

Fig. 9. A patient with pain 2 years after lumbar spine fusion surgery. MIP image (*A*) and sagittal fused image (*B*) show an endplate fracture of the first lumbar vertebral body with markedly increased ^{18}F NaF uptake (*arrow*). In addition, there is increased uptake (*arrowhead*) around the cage L5/S1, indicating microinstability and incomplete incorporation of the implant.

[18]F NaF uptake. The investigators concluded that this finding might be a sign of microinstability and, thus, missing/incomplete osseous fusion.

Condylar Hyperplasia

Imaging with bone-seeking radiopharmaceuticals can be helpful in patients with condylar hyperplasia or hemimandibular elongation, to assess the growth activity of the mandibular condyle and to guide the treatment. BS with SPECT is an established imaging tool with quantification of the side difference.[44,45] Laverick and colleagues[46] used [18]F NaF PET/CT instead of ^{99m}Tc-MDP SPECT/CT in 5 patients who were suspected of having condylar hyperplasia, and the results were correlated with the operative findings. The technique correctly identified condylar hyperplasia in all patients. The investigators concluded that [18]F NaF PET is a valid method of assessing patients with condylar hyperplasia.

SUMMARY

Preliminary data and experience with [18]F NaF PET/CT in benign bone disease are promising. Some clinical situations including insufficiency fractures, occult fractures, osteoarthritis, osteoid osteoma, failed back surgery, and child abuse are auspicious indications for [18]F NaF PET/CT imaging. It is also useful for the evaluation of bone metabolism in diseases such as osteoporosis.

With developments in PET technology, more availability of PET/CT machines, and routine performance of dynamic quantitative imaging, [18]F NaF PET/CT will probably play a major role in the assessment of various benign bone diseases in the near future. However, further comparative studies are needed with larger patient numbers and direct comparison with established imaging modalities such as ^{99m}Tc-MDP SPECT/CT, SPECT/CT, and morphologic imaging (eg, MR imaging).

REFERENCES

1. Gould P. Medical isotope shortage reaches crisis level. Nature 2009;460(7253):312–3.
2. Even-Sapir E, Metser U, Mishani E, et al. The detection of bone metastases in patients with high-risk prostate cancer: ^{99m}Tc-MDP planar bone scintigraphy, single- and multi-field-of-view SPECT, ^{18}F-fluoride PET, and ^{18}F-fluoride PET/CT. J Nucl Med 2006;47(2):287–97.
3. Piert M, Zittel TT, Becker GA, et al. Assessment of porcine bone metabolism by dynamic. J Nucl Med 2001;42(7):1091–100.
4. Messa C, Goodman WG, Hoh CK, et al. Bone metabolic activity measured with positron emission tomography and [^{18}F]fluoride ion in renal osteodystrophy: correlation with bone histomorphometry. J Clin Endocrinol Metab 1993;77(4):949–55.
5. Uchida K, Nakajima H, Miyazaki T, et al. Effects of alendronate on bone metabolism in glucocorticoid-induced osteoporosis measured by ^{18}F-fluoride PET: a prospective study. J Nucl Med 2009;50(11):1808–14.
6. Song IH, Carrasco-Fernandez J, Rudwaleit M, et al. The diagnostic value of scintigraphy in assessing sacroiliitis in ankylosing spondylitis: a systematic literature research. Ann Rheum Dis 2008;67(11):1535–40.
7. Battafarano DF, West SG, Rak KM, et al. Comparison of bone scan, computed tomography, and magnetic resonance imaging in the diagnosis of active sacroiliitis. Semin Arthritis Rheum 1993;23(3):161–76.
8. Blum U, Buitrago-Tellez C, Mundinger A, et al. Magnetic resonance imaging (MRI) for detection of active sacroiliitis—a prospective study comparing conventional radiography, scintigraphy, and contrast enhanced MRI. J Rheumatol 1996;23(12):2107–15.
9. Strobel K, Fischer DR, Tamborrini G, et al. ^{18}F-fluoride PET/CT for detection of sacroiliitis in ankylosing spondylitis. Eur J Nucl Med Mol Imaging 2010;37(9):1760–5.
10. Czernin J, Satyamurthy N, Schiepers C. Molecular mechanisms of bone ^{18}F-NaF deposition. J Nucl Med 2010;51(12):1826–9.
11. Li Y, Schiepers C, Lake R, et al. Clinical utility of (18)F-fluoride PET/CT in benign and malignant bone diseases. Bone 2012;50(1):128–39.
12. Weber U, Pfirrmann CW, Kissling RO, et al. Whole body MR imaging in ankylosing spondylitis: a descriptive pilot study in patients with suspected early and active confirmed ankylosing spondylitis. BMC Musculoskelet Disord 2007;8:20.
13. Fischer DR, Pfirrmann CW, Zubler V, et al. High bone turnover assessed by ^{18}F-fluoride PET/CT in the spine of patients with ankylosing spondylitis: no redundancy to inflammatory lesions detected by whole body MRI. Abstract EULAR 2012.
14. Baraliakos X, Listing J, Brandt J, et al. Radiographic progression in patients with ankylosing spondylitis after 4 yrs of treatment with the anti-TNF-alpha antibody infliximab. Rheumatology (Oxford) 2007;46(9):1450–3.
15. Drubach LA, Johnston PR, Newton AW, et al. Skeletal trauma in child abuse: detection with ^{18}F-NaF PET. Radiology 2010;255(1):173–81.
16. Dua SG, Purandare NC, Shah S, et al. F-18 fluoride PET/CT in the detection of radiation-induced pelvic insufficiency fractures. Clin Nucl Med 2011;36(10):e146–9.

17. Love C, Tomas MB, Marwin SE, et al. Role of nuclear medicine in diagnosis of the infected joint replacement. Radiographics 2001;21(5):1229–38.

18. Hirschmann MT, Davda K, Rasch H, et al. Clinical value of combined single photon emission computerized tomography and conventional computer tomography (SPECT/CT) in sports medicine. Sports Med Arthrosc 2011;19(2):174–81.

19. Hirschmann MT, Konala P, Iranpour F, et al. Clinical value of SPECT/CT for evaluation of patients with painful knees after total knee arthroplasty—a new dimension of diagnostics? BMC Musculoskelet Disord 2011;12:36.

20. Kobayashi N, Inaba Y, Choe H, et al. Use of F-18 fluoride PET to differentiate septic from aseptic loosening in total hip arthroplasty patients. Clin Nucl Med 2011;36(11):e156–61.

21. Choe H, Inaba Y, Kobayashi N, et al. Use of ^{18}F-fluoride PET to determine the appropriate tissue sampling region for improved sensitivity of tissue examinations in cases of suspected periprosthetic infection after total hip arthroplasty. Acta Orthop 2011;82(4):427–32.

22. Sterner T, Pink R, Freudenberg L, et al. The role of [^{18}F]fluoride positron emission tomography in the early detection of aseptic loosening of total knee arthroplasty. Int J Surg 2007;5(2):99–104.

23. Rajender K, Rakesh K, Suhas S, et al. Role of ^{18}F-fluoride PET/CT and ^{18}F FDG PET/CT for differentiating septic from aseptic loosening in patients with painful hip prosthesis. J Nucl Med 2011;52(Suppl 1):458.

24. Zoccali C, Teori G, Salducca N. The role of FDG-PET in distinguishing between septic and aseptic loosening in hip prosthesis: a review of literature. Int Orthop 2009;33(1):1–5.

25. Stumpe KD, Notzli HP, Zanetti M, et al. FDG PET for differentiation of infection and aseptic loosening in total hip replacements: comparison with conventional radiography and three-phase bone scintigraphy. Radiology 2004;231(2):333–41.

26. Love C, Marwin SE, Tomas MB, et al. Diagnosing infection in the failed joint replacement: a comparison of coincidence detection ^{18}F-FDG and ^{111}In-labeled leukocyte/^{99m}Tc-sulfur colloid marrow imaging. J Nucl Med 2004;45(11):1864–71.

27. Grant FD, Fahey FH, Packard AB, et al. Skeletal PET with ^{18}F-fluoride: applying new technology to an old tracer. J Nucl Med 2008;49(1):68–78.

28. Farid K, El-Deeb G, Caillat Vigneron N. SPECT-CT improves scintigraphic accuracy of osteoid osteoma diagnosis. Clin Nucl Med 2010;35(3):170–1.

29. Assoun J, Richardi G, Railhac JJ, et al. Osteoid osteoma: MR imaging versus CT. Radiology 1994;191(1):217–23.

30. Even-Sapir E, Mishani E, Flusser G, et al. ^{18}F-Fluoride positron emission tomography and positron emission tomography/computed tomography. Semin Nucl Med 2007;37(6):462–9.

31. Wilde F, Steinhoff K, Frerich B, et al. Positron-emission tomography imaging in the diagnosis of bisphosphonate-related osteonecrosis of the jaw. Oral Surg Oral Med Oral Pathol Oral Radiol Endod 2009;107(3):412–9.

32. Hakim SG, Bruecker CW, Jacobsen H, et al. The value of FDG-PET and bone scintigraphy with SPECT in the primary diagnosis and follow-up of patients with chronic osteomyelitis of the mandible. Int J Oral Maxillofac Surg 2006;35(9):809–16.

33. Dasa V, Adbel-Nabi H, Anders MJ, et al. F-18 fluoride positron emission tomography of the hip for osteonecrosis. Clin Orthop Relat Res 2008;466(5):1081–6.

34. Brenner W, Vernon C, Conrad EU, et al. Assessment of the metabolic activity of bone grafts with (18)F-fluoride PET. Eur J Nucl Med Mol Imaging 2004;31(9):1291–8.

35. Berding G, Schliephake H, van den Hoff J, et al. Assessment of the incorporation of revascularized fibula grafts used for mandibular reconstruction with F-18-PET. Nuklearmedizin 2001;40(2):51–8.

36. Piert M, Winter E, Becker GA, et al. Allogenic bone graft viability after hip revision arthroplasty assessed by dynamic [^{18}F]fluoride ion positron emission tomography. Eur J Nucl Med 1999;26(6):615–24.

37. Sörensen J, Michaelsson K, Strand H, et al. Longstanding increased bone turnover at the fixation points after anterior cruciate ligament reconstruction: a positron emission tomography (PET) study of 8 patients. Acta Orthop 2006;77(6):921–5.

38. Fischer DR, Maquieira GJ, Espinosa N, et al. Therapeutic impact of [(18)F]fluoride positron-emission tomography/computed tomography on patients with unclear foot pain. Skeletal Radiol 2010;39(10):987–97.

39. Pagenstert GI, Barg A, Leumann AG, et al. SPECT-CT imaging in degenerative joint disease of the foot and ankle. J Bone Joint Surg Br 2009;91(9):1191–6.

40. Samarin A, Fischer D, Betz M, et al. Clinical relevance of 18-fluoride uptake in PET/CT in the asymptomatic and symptomatic foot. Abstract RSNA 2011.

41. Ovadia D, Metser U, Lievshitz G, et al. Back pain in adolescents: assessment with integrated ^{18}F-fluoride positron-emission tomography-computed tomography. J Pediatr Orthop 2007;27(1):90–3.

42. Lim R, Fahey FH, Drubach LA, et al. Early experience with fluorine-18 sodium fluoride bone PET in young patients with back pain. J Pediatr Orthop 2007;27(3):277–82.

43. Fischer DR, Zweifel K, Treyer V, et al. Assessment of successful incorporation of cages after cervical or lumbar intercorporeal fusion with [(18)F]fluoride positron-emission tomography/computed tomography. Eur Spine J 2011;20(4):640–8.

44. Saridin CP, Raijmakers P, Becking AG. Quantitative analysis of planar bone scintigraphy in patients with unilateral condylar hyperplasia. Oral Surg Oral Med Oral Pathol Oral Radiol Endod 2007;104(2):259–63.

45. Saridin CP, Raijmakers PG, Tuinzing DB, et al. Comparison of planar bone scintigraphy and single photon emission computed tomography in patients suspected of having unilateral condylar hyperactivity. Oral Surg Oral Med Oral Pathol Oral Radiol Endod 2008;106(3):426–32.

46. Laverick S, Bounds G, Wong WL. [^{18}F]-fluoride positron emission tomography for imaging condylar hyperplasia. Br J Oral Maxillofac Surg 2009;47(3): 196–9.

^{18}F NaF PET/CT in the Assessment of Malignant Bone Disease

Camila Mosci, MD, Andrei Iagaru, MD*

KEYWORDS

- ^{18}F NaF PET/CT • Malignant bone disease • Primary bone cancer • Bone metastasis

KEY POINTS

- ^{18}F-Labeled sodium fluoride (^{18}F NaF) is a positron-emitting radiopharmaceutical with desirable characteristics (rapid blood clearance and bone uptake) for high-quality functional imaging of the skeleton.
- ^{18}F NaF PET/computed tomography (CT) is able to detect osseous lesions with improved results (higher sensitivity and specificity) when compared with ^{99m}Tc–methylene diphosphonate (^{99m}Tc-MDP) planar and single-photon emission CT bone scintigraphy.
- ^{18}F NaF PET/CT allows for shorter imaging time, thus improving patients' convenience and benefiting the overall workflow of the imaging facility.
- ^{18}F NaF PET/CT can be used to evaluate both primary bone cancers and bone metastases accurately.
- Future clinical trials required for the validation of preliminary reports on ^{18}F NaF imaging of the skeleton are very likely to be conducted using novel technologies such as the combined and simultaneous PET and magnetic resonance imaging whole-body scanners.

INTRODUCTION

^{18}F-Labeled sodium fluoride (^{18}F NaF) is a positron-emitting radiopharmaceutical that was used briefly for skeletal scintigraphy in the 1970s. Its clinical use was limited at that time because of the logistic difficulties in delivering a tracer with a half-life of 109.74 minutes, as well as the less than ideal features of conventional gamma cameras. ^{18}F NaF was largely replaced in the late 1970s by ^{99m}Tc-labeled diphosphonates, which have optimal characteristics for conventional gamma cameras.[1,2] ^{18}F NaF is an avid bone seeker, a property attributable to it being an analogue of the hydroxyl group found in the hydroxyapatite bone crystals. Ion exchange is the mechanism of uptake for ^{18}F NaF, and blood flow is probably the rate-limiting step in the transfer of fluoride ions from blood to bone.[3] As with ^{99m}Tc-based bone agents, which adhere to bone by chemical absorption, fluorine is directly incorporated into the bone matrix, converting hydroxyapatite to fluoroapatite.[4] ^{18}F NaF is rapidly cleared from the plasma, as it has a smaller proportion that is protein bound in comparison with ^{99m}Tc–methylene diphosphonate (^{99m}Tc-MDP), and is excreted by the kidneys, with first-pass extraction approaching 100%.[5] One hour after injection, only 10% of ^{18}F NaF remains in the plasma.[1] Its desirable characteristics of high and rapid bone uptake, accompanied by very rapid blood clearance, result in a high bone-to-background ratio in a short time. High-quality images of the skeleton can be obtained less than 1 hour after the intravenous administration of ^{18}F NaF. The nonuniform pattern of

Division of Nuclear Medicine, Stanford University Medical Center, 300 Pasteur Drive, H-2200, Stanford, CA 94305-5281, USA
* Corresponding author.
E-mail address: aiagaru@stanford.edu

PET Clin 7 (2012) 263–274
doi:10.1016/j.cpet.2012.04.003
1556-8598/12/$ – see front matter © 2012 Elsevier Inc. All rights reserved.

uptake seen in the distribution of ^{18}F NaF in the normal skeleton reflects differences in regional blood flow as well as nonuniformity in the accessibility to the bone crystal surface. Areas of high uptake in abnormal scans result from any processes that increase the exposed bone crystal surface and/or the blood flow. Areas of osteolytic activity can be visualized just as well as areas of osteoblastic activity.[3]

^{18}F NAF PET/CT VERSUS ^{99M}TC-MDP BONE SCINTIGRAPHY

Efforts currently under way in the molecular imaging community aim to provide sound scientific data regarding the benefits of using ^{18}F NaF PET/computed tomography (CT) for detection of malignant skeletal lesions.[6] The Centers for Medicare and Medicaid Services (CMS) issued a decision memorandum regarding the use of ^{18}F NaF PET for detection of bony metastasis in February 2010, concluding that the available evidence was sufficient to allow coverage for ^{18}F NaF PET under coverage with evidence development. This decision resulted in the creation of the National Oncologic PET Registry for ^{18}F NaF (NOPR [NaF PET]).[7] ^{99m}Tc-MDP bone scintigraphy has been the method of choice for evaluation of osseous metastases in various cancers, because it allows a whole-body survey at relatively low cost. Successful imaging of skeletal metastases is achieved for prostate, lung, breast, and other cancers.[8] Applications of skeletal scintigraphy include initial staging, monitoring the response to therapy, and detection of areas at risk for pathologic fracture. Although ^{99m}Tc-MDP scintigraphy is sensitive for the detection of advanced skeletal metastatic lesions, early involvement may be missed because this technique relies on the identification of the osteoblastic reaction of the involved bone rather than the detection of the tumor itself. The technique also relies significantly on the regional blood flow to bone. Limitations imposed by the spatial resolution of planar scintigraphy and single-photon emission CT (SPECT) also affect the sensitivity of bone scintigraphy in the detection of osseous metastases.[9]

Thus, the transition to the better resolution of PET/CT for detection of osseous metastases is appealing, with the use of the positron emitter ^{18}F NaF as the radiotracer of choice. Recent studies compared ^{18}F NaF PET to ^{99m}Tc-MDP scintigraphy,[10–13] and showed that ^{18}F NaF PET is more accurate than ^{99m}Tc-MDP planar imaging or SPECT for localizing and characterizing malignant bone lesions. The higher-quality imaging, increased clinical accuracy, greater convenience to the patient and referring physician, and more efficient use of nuclear medicine resources all indicate the need to reconsider the use of ^{18}F NaF PET for imaging malignant diseases of the skeleton.[10] Despite the high performance of ^{18}F NaF PET/CT, its clinical use remains limited because there are fewer PET/CT scanners than gamma cameras, and its utility is related to the lack of uniform reimbursement practices.

PRIMARY BONE TUMORS

Primary bone tumors are very rare neoplasms that occur mainly in pediatric patients and young adults, accounting for approximately 5% of childhood malignancies and 0.2% of all primary cancers in adults.[14] The etiology remains unclear, but genetic alterations and radiation therapy have been described as one of the factors.[15] In 2012 an estimated 2890 new cases will be diagnosed in the United States, and 1410 people will die from primary bone cancers.[16] The factors potentially responsible for poorer outcomes are multiple and include delayed diagnosis, tumor biology, and complex challenges related to chemotherapy administration.[17] The diagnosis of primary bone cancer is usually associated with a poor prognosis, but the development of novel diagnostic methods and treatment algorithms has resulted in improvements in survival, particularly for early-stage disease. Staging is therefore important for prognosis and to define the proper therapy. The National Comprehensive Cancer Network Clinical Practice Guidelines suggest that both the American Joint Committee on Cancer (AJCC) system and the Surgical Staging System (SSS) should be used for osteosarcoma staging. The AJCC is based on the assessment of histologic grade (G), and presence of regional (N) and distant metastases (M). The SSS is based on the surgical grade (G), local extent (T), and presence of regional and distant metastases.[15] Considering the historical perspective given by the prior use of ^{99m}Tc-MDP bone scintigraphy in the management of malignant primary bone lesions, ^{18}F NaF PET/CT has the potential to play an important role in the grading, staging, and evaluation of response to therapy in primary bone tumors.

Osteosarcoma

Osteosarcoma is the most common malignant primary bone tumor, accounting for 35% of bone tumors.[18] The peak of incidence is the second decade of life. Osteosarcomas are classified into intramedullary, surface, and extraskeletal. High-grade intramedullary osteosarcoma is the most common, accounting for approximately 80%. Osteosarcoma most commonly affects metaphyseal areas in the distal femur and proximal tibia (sites of maximum growth), followed by proximal femur, proximal humerus, and jaw.[19] Significant prognostic factors are tumor size and site, presence and location of metastases, and response to chemotherapy. Accurate imaging of osteosarcoma is important for clinical staging and monitoring response to therapy. Plain radiographs and magnetic resonance (MR) imaging are used for the accurate evaluation of the primary lesion. In addition, ^{99m}Tc-MDP bone scintigraphy is used for the detection of skip lesions.[15] Although ^{18}F-fluorodeoxyglucose (^{18}F-FDG) PET/CT has a limited role in the diagnosis of osteosarcoma, several reports suggest that it is suitable for staging, prognostication, and evaluation of therapy response.[15,20–23]

The utility of [18]F NaF PET and [18]F NaF PET/CT in the management of osteosarcoma has been evaluated in preliminary reports, usually with small number of participants included. An early study was published by Hoh and colleagues[24] on the use of [18]F NaF for PET imaging of the skeleton. Among 13 patients with documented malignant bone lesions, 4 had osteosarcoma. When compared with other malignant bone lesions, untreated osteosarcoma had the highest tumor-to-normal bone activity ratios. The investigators also reported that in one patient the tumor activity was notably reduced after treatment with chemotherapy and immunotherapy. This finding suggests that quantitative [18]F NaF PET/CT may also be useful for monitoring therapy response, including the response to neoadjuvant chemotherapy before surgical resection. Based on its mechanism of bone uptake, [18]F NaF PET/CT may also allow the detection of viable, nonnecrotic and, thus, chemotherapy-resistant parts of the tumor, possibly predicting prognosis.

Similarly to reports on ^{99m}Tc-MDP bone scintigraphy, increased [18]F NaF uptake has been noted in patients with proven lung metastases from osteosarcoma.[25] Although chest CT is the method of choice for detecting pulmonary metastases, [18]F NaF PET may have a unique potential when compared with ^{18}F-FDG in detecting metastases to the lungs or secondary bone lesions for both primary staging and restaging purposes.[26] This aspect is particularly important, given that several studies demonstrated that pulmonary metastases from osteosarcomas and Ewing sarcomas tend to not be ^{18}F-FDG avid, regardless of size.[27–29]

Ewing Sarcoma

Ewing sarcoma is the third most common malignant bone tumor, accounting for approximately 16%.[15] Similarly to osteosarcomas, the pathogenesis and etiology seem to be related to gene rearrangements.[15] It is slightly more common in males (male/female ratio of 55:45).[30] The most common age of diagnosis is the second decade of life, although 20% to 30% of cases are diagnosed in the first decade and some cases are diagnosed through the third decade.[30] In Ewing sarcoma, increasing age has consistently been demonstrated to be associated with a poorer prognosis. The most common sites of primary Ewing sarcoma are the pelvic bones, the long bones of the lower extremities, and the bones of the chest wall. As opposed to osteosarcoma, they tend to arise from the diaphyseal rather than the metaphyseal portion of the bone. The most common site of metastases are the lungs, bone, and bone marrow; these are detectable in about 25% of patients.[30] Locoregional lymph node involvement is rare. Clinical symptoms include localized pain and/or swelling, but symptoms such as fever, weight loss, and fatigue can occasionally be noted at presentation. In the past, fewer than 10% of patients survived, and patients would die from metastatic disease within 2 years. However, with development of better diagnostic methods and treatment, survival rates have improved, particularly in patients with localized disease.[15]

Imaging studies should include CT scan of the chest to document or exclude intrathoracic metastases and ^{99m}Tc-MDP bone scintigraphy to evaluate for skeletal metastases. ^{18}F-FDG PET has been proposed as a sensitive method for the definition of extent of disease in Ewing sarcoma, although its exact role in its management remains to be defined.[31,32] Moreover, the initial response to neoadjuvant chemotherapy as shown by changes in the standardized uptake value (SUV) may predict outcome.[30] Given the low incidence of Ewing sarcoma, there are no published reports on the use of [18]F NaF. However, in the authors' experience, such lesions tend to demonstrate intense [18]F NaF, as is illustrated in **Fig. 1**.

MULTIPLE MYELOMA

Multiple myeloma (MM) is a neoplastic proliferation of plasma cells within the bone marrow. MM has an unknown etiology and affects the elderly (median age at diagnosis 70 years). MM is twice as common in African Americans as in Caucasians, and there is a slight male preponderance. The American Cancer Society estimates that the number of new cases and deaths caused by MM in 2012 will be 21,700 and 10,710, respectively.[16] Prognosis for the disease is highly variable, with survival ranging from a few months to more than 10 years.[33]

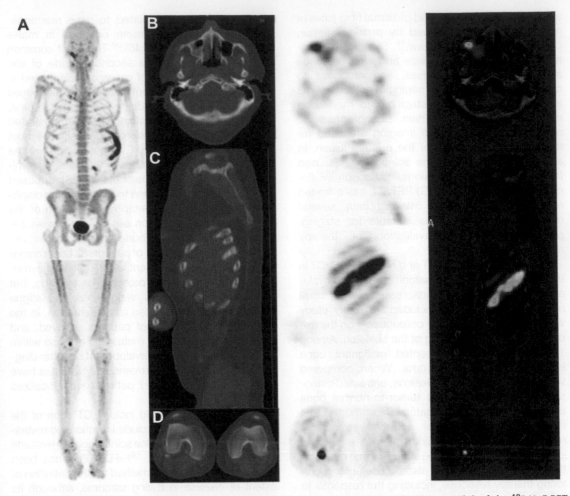

Fig. 1. A 22-year-old man with Ewing sarcoma. Maximum-intensity projection (MIP) image (*A*) of the ^{18}F NaF PET shows several regions of increased uptake, corresponding to maxillary sinus uptake related to inflammation (*B*), the primary Ewing sarcoma rib lesion (*C*), and benign muscle calcification (*D*). CT, PET, and fused PET/CT images are shown.

Clinical presentation includes fatigue, anemia, or recurrent infection due to bone marrow infiltration, bone pain, pathologic fractures, and renal failure. However, up to 20% of cases of MM are asymptomatic and found incidentally. Diagnosis of MM is made through the detection in blood and/or urine of a monoclonal protein produced by the abnormal plasma cells. Once the diagnosis is suspected, a radiographic skeletal survey, bone marrow aspiration, and biopsy are conducted to confirm the diagnosis and evaluate the extent of disease.[33] The characteristic bone lesion is seen as a sharply defined small lytic area with no reactive bone formation arising in the medulla; the absence of bone sclerosis is due to inhibition of osteoblastic activity.[34] The most commonly affected sites are the vertebrae (66% of cases), ribs (45%), skull (40%), and pelvis (30%).[35] The skeletal survey includes a series of plain films of the chest, skull, humerus, femur, pelvis, and spine. Bone scintigraphy with ^{99m}Tc-MDP has a limited role in staging MM because of the lack of radiotracer uptake in the lytic lesions. Its sensitivity in detecting MM bone disease was found to range between 40% and 60%.[36]

Features of an optimal imaging technique include high sensitivity for detecting lytic bone lesions, infiltrative lesions in the bone marrow, and extramedullary disease, as well as being able to assess response to treatment. ^{18}F NaF PET/CT has the potential to detect lesions, provide prognosis, and evaluate response to treatment in MM. Its role in MM is currently evaluated in several ongoing research trials, but preliminary reports indicate that the potential for quantitation makes ^{18}F NaF PET/CT an attractive alternative to conventional bone scanning.[37] An example of ^{18}F NaF PET/CT in a patient diagnosed with MM is presented in **Fig. 2.**

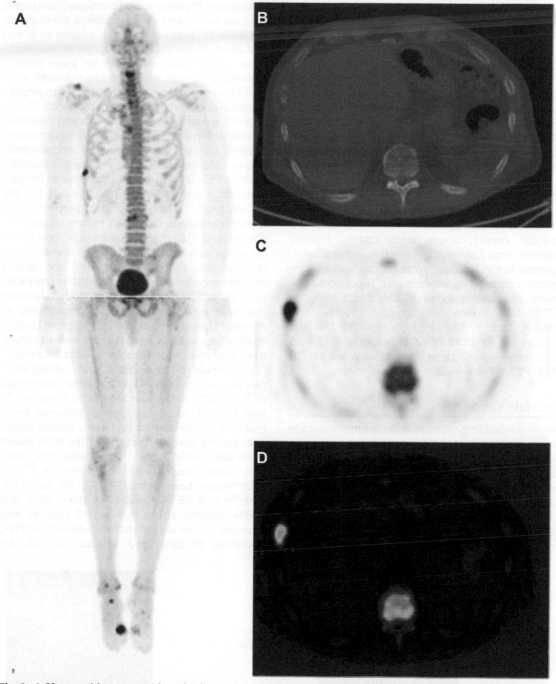

Fig. 2. A 60-year-old woman with multiple myeloma. MIP image (*A*) of the ¹⁸F NaF PET shows increased uptake in a rib, viewed in detail on transaxial CT (*B*), PET (*C*), and fused PET/CT (*D*).

BONE METASTASES

Imaging modalities have a major role in the evaluation of patients with suspected bone metastases. Currently used methods include ⁹⁹ᵐTc-MDP bone scintigraphy, CT, MR imaging, and more recently, combined functional and anatomic imaging using PET/CT. PET/CT evaluation of the skeleton can be performed with different tracers, including ¹⁸F NaF and ¹⁸F-FDG.

Even-Sapir and colleagues[38] evaluated ¹⁸F NaF PET/CT in 44 patients with cancer. In this group there were subjects with various types of cancers: breast, prostate, lung, colon, nasopharynx, testes, gastrointestinal, lymphoma, melanoma, MM, sarcoma, giant-cell tumor, and carcinoid. The PET/CT was indicated for surveillance, pain investigation, and suspicion of bone involvement derived from abnormal laboratory findings or unclear findings on other imaging modalities. In patient-based analysis the investigators reported a sensitivity of 88% for PET alone and 100% for PET/CT. Specificity was 56% and 88% for PET and PET/CT, respectively. This report also indicated that [18]F NaF PET/CT accurately differentiates malignant from benign bone lesions.

[18]F NaF PET/CT and ^{18}F-FDG PET/CT were compared for the evaluation of skeletal metastases in another study.[13] The patient population was also heterogeneous: sarcoma, prostate cancer, breast cancer, colon cancer, bladder cancer, lung cancer, paraganglioma, lymphoma, gastrointestinal cancer, renal cancer, and salivary gland cancer. The investigators reported sensitivity and specificity of 87.5% and 92.9% for ^{99m}Tc-MDP bone scintigraphy, 95.8% and 92.9% for [18]F NaF PET/CT, and 66.7% and 96.4% for ^{18}F FDG PET/CT, respectively. **Fig. 3** presents sclerotic bone metastases noted on [18]F NaF PET/CT in a patient with renal cancer.

Prostate Cancer

Prostate cancer is the most common malignancy in men, accounting for 29% of all tumors, and the second cause of cancer-related deaths in the same population. The American Cancer Society estimates 241,740 new cases of prostate cancer and 28,170 deaths attributable to it in 2012.[16] Prostate cancer ranges from asymptomatic to rapidly progressive systemic malignancy, and lymph nodes and bones are the most common sites of metastases. Prostate-specific antigen (PSA) levels, Gleason score, and clinical stage at presentation are used for pretreatment risk assessment, and evaluation of the probability for local recurrence or metastatic disease. Based on these criteria, patients are characterized as low risk (unlikely to have bone metastases) and high risk. Thus, skeletal metastases are related to a poor prognosis. ^{99m}Tc-MDP bone scans have been the imaging method of choice for the evaluation of skeletal metastases in prostate cancer because they are predominantly sclerotic. Advanced molecular imaging modalities such as PET/CT may assist conventional imaging methods. Several studies have reported a low sensitivity of ^{18}F-FDG PET for the detection of prostate cancer lesions. Other PET tracers such as ^{18}F-choline and ^{11}C-choline have been reported to have high sensitivity in detecting local recurrence, regional lymph node involvement, and distant involvement after radical prostatectomy and radiation therapy.[39] [18]F NaF PET/CT, although still being evaluated in research projects,[40] may have an important role in the detection of malignant skeletal involvement in both pretreatment and posttreatment scenarios in patients with prostate cancer.[41]

In a study by Even-Sapir and colleagues,[10] patients with a high risk of prostate cancer had a ^{99m}Tc-MDP bone scan with SPECT and an [18]F NaF PET/CT scan. Comparison between these methods demonstrated that on a patient-based analysis the sensitivity of the ^{99m}Tc-MDP planar bone scan, SPECT, and [18]F NaF was 70%, 92%, and 100%, respectively. Specificity of ^{99m}Tc-MDP planar bone scan, SPECT, [18]F NaF PET, and [18]F NaF PET/CT was 57%, 82%, 62%, and 100%. Another study involving 42 patients with prostate cancer demonstrated sensitivity of 91%, specificity of 89%, and accuracy of 90% for

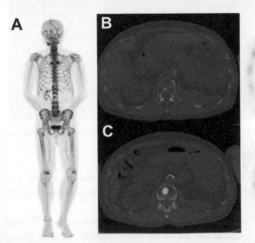
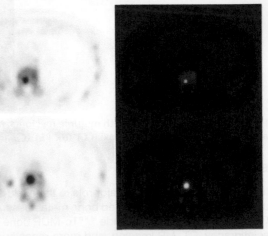

Fig. 3. A 65-year-old man with renal cancer. MIP image (*A*) of the [18]F NaF PET shows increased uptake in 2 lumbar vertebrae sclerotic metastases, viewed in detail on transaxial CT, PET, and fused PET/CT (*B, C*).

^{18}F NaF PET/CT in the detection of bone metastases.[42] **Fig. 4** shows ^{18}F NaF–avid bone metastases in a patient with prostate cancer.

^{18}F NaF PET/CT may also play an important role in monitoring treatment response in prostate cancer. Cook and colleagues[43] compared qualitative bone scintigraphy with semiquantitative ^{18}F-NaF PET for the evaluation of response to bone metastases treatment with ^{223}Ra-chloride. The investigators concluded that ^{18}F NaF PET is more accurate than ^{99m}Tc-MDP bone scintigraphy.

Breast Cancer

Breast cancer is the most common malignancy in women. The American Cancer Society estimated that 226,870 new cases of invasive breast cancer would be diagnosed in the United States in 2012 and that 39,510 patients would die of the disease.[16] The incidence of breast cancer has increased over the past few decades, but mortality seems to be declining, suggesting a benefit from early detection, development of imaging methods, and more effective treatment.

The most common site of metastases from breast cancer is the skeleton. These lesions are predominantly osteolytic, but 15% to 20% of patients can present osteoblastic lesions.[44] It has been demonstrated that the distribution of metastatic bone lesions is an important prognostic factor. In a study comprising 82 patients, Yamashita and colleagues[45] suggested that the distribution of metastatic bone lesions on the bone scan

and the presence of radiographic osteosclerosis in metastatic bone lesions should be considered prognostic variables for patients with breast cancer and metastasis confined initially to bone. Therefore, ^{18}F NaF PET may play an important prognostic role in these patients. Multiple bone metastases are noted on the ^{18}F NaF PET/CT scan in a patient with breast cancer presented in **Fig. 5**.

Petrn-Mallmin and colleagues[46] investigated how the areas of pathologic uptake of ^{18}F NaF seen on PET relate to bone structure on CT. For this purpose both visual analysis of the radionuclide uptake and analysis of the skeletal kinetics of the ^{18}F NaF with dynamic PET imaging were performed in patients with skeletal metastases from breast cancer. The lytic, sclerotic, and mixed lesions found on CT all corresponded to areas with an increased uptake of ^{18}F NaF on PET. The exceptions were small lytic lesions, 2 to 3 mm in size, which were not identified on PET. Moreover, the investigators noticed no difference in the uptake of ^{18}F NaF between lytic and sclerotic lesions. Both lytic and sclerotic lesions had markedly higher uptake than normal bone (5–10 times higher).

Although ^{99m}Tc-MDP bone scanning, CT, and MR imaging can detect skeletal metastases from breast cancer, the evaluation of response to treatment of bone metastasis is difficult to assess using these conventional modalities. It has been proposed that ^{18}F NaF PET may be useful for assessing changes in bone turnover in response to

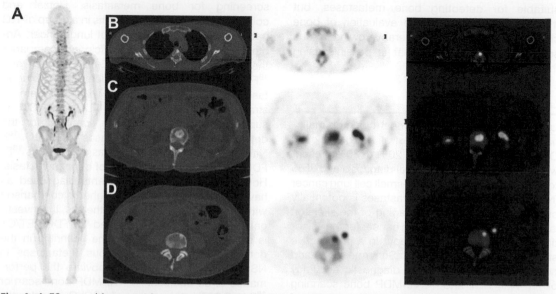

Fig. 4. A 58-year-old man with prostate cancer. MIP image (*A*) of the ^{18}F NaF PET shows increased uptake in multiple osseous metastases, viewed in detail on transaxial CT, PET and fused PET/CT (*B–D*).

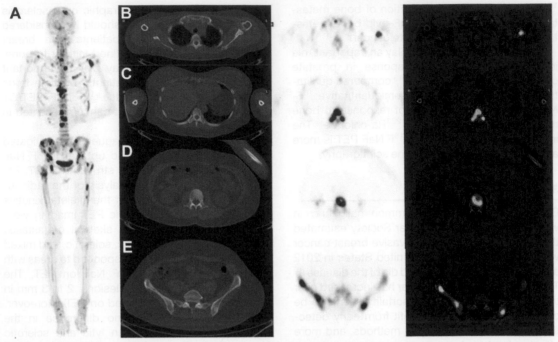

Fig. 5. A 72-year-old woman with breast cancer. MIP image (*A*) of the ^{18}F NaF PET shows increased uptake in multiple osseous metastases, viewed in detail on transaxial CT, PET, and fused PET/CT (*B–E*).

therapy. Doot and colleagues[47] used dynamic ^{18}F NaF PET to characterize the fluoride kinetics of bone metastases in patients with breast cancer, and found that ^{18}F NaF transport (K_1) and flux (K_i) were significantly different in metastases and normal bone. The investigators also stated that these values could be estimated with reasonable precision and accuracy. ^{18}F NaF PET is not only suitable for detecting bone metastases, but may also be useful for the evaluation of bone changes in response to therapy, owing to the semiquantitative analysis that is possible using this approach.

Lung Cancer

Lung cancer is the second most common malignancy, accounting for 14% of all malignancies.[16] Of patients with lung cancer, 20% to 30% present with bone metastases at initial diagnosis and 35% to 60% at autopsy.[48–50] Non–small cell lung cancer (NSCLC) without distant metastases is potentially curable. Hence, accurate staging of the skeleton is crucial in patients with lung cancer for the selection of the appropriate therapy. In a prospective study of 53 patients, Schirrmeister and colleagues[51] compared the diagnostic accuracy of ^{18}F NaF PET and ^{99m}Tc-MDP bone scanning with and without SPECT at the initial staging of lung cancer. In this group of patients, 12 had

bone metastases. There were 6 false negatives on the ^{99m}Tc-MDP bone scan, 1 on SPECT, and none on ^{18}F NaF PET. ^{99m}Tc-MDP SPECT and ^{18}F NaF PET changed clinical management in 5 patients (9%) and 6 patients (11%), respectively. The investigators concluded that although SPECT improves the accuracy of bone scan, PET is the most accurate whole-body imaging modality for screening for bone metastasis. Hetzel and colleagues[52] found similar results in a group of 103 patients with initial diagnosis of lung cancer. Another study involving 126 participants compared the diagnostic accuracy of ^{18}F-FDG PET/CT and ^{18}F NaF PET/CT for the detection of bone metastases in patients with NSCLC. This study demonstrated that integrated ^{18}F-FDG PET/CT is superior to ^{99m}Tc-MDP bone scanning for the detection of osteolytic metastases in NSCLC. ^{18}F NaF PET seems to be at least as sensitive as ^{18}F-FDG PET/CT for the detection of bone metastasis. However, the number of patients diagnosed as having bone metastasis was higher in comparison with ^{18}F-FDG PET/CT.[11] Nevertheless, the investigators concluded that integrated ^{18}F-FDG PET/CT is superior to ^{99m}Tc-MDP bone scanning in the detection of osteolytic osseous metastases in NSCLC, and therefore may obviate the performance of an additional ^{99m}Tc-MDP bone scan or ^{18}F NaF PET in the staging of NSCLC, significantly reducing costs.

FUTURE DIRECTIONS

Combining ^{18}F NaF and ^{18}F-FDG in a single PET/CT scan for evaluation of malignant skeletal disease may result in a more convenient schedule for the patient, less radiation, and potential savings in health care costs. Instead of patients having to undergo separate PET/CT studies, usually on different days, this strategy allows for one combined PET/CT study. The preliminary results of a prospective, international multicenter trial proved the feasibility of combined administration of ^{18}F NaF and ^{18}F-FDG in a single PET/CT examination for detection of malignancy.[53–55] **Fig. 6**

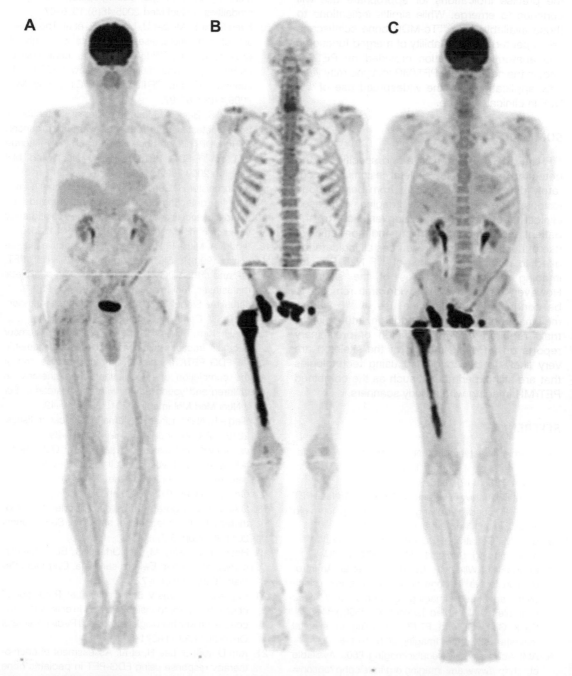

Fig. 6. A 74-year-old man with metastatic prostate cancer. Extensive pelvic osseous metastases are not identified on the ^{18}F-FDG PET (A), but are clearly seen on the ^{18}F NaF (B) and combined (C) PET scans.

shows maximum-intensity projection images from a patient with prostate cancer. Extensive pelvic osseous metastases are not identified on the ^{18}F-FDG PET scan (see **Fig. 6**A), but are clearly seen on the ^{18}F NaF (see **Fig. 6**B) and combined (see **Fig. 6**C) PET scans.

As more imaging centers begin using ^{18}F NaF routinely for PET/CT evaluation of the skeleton, the precise indications for appropriate use will continue to emerge. While similar indications to those available for ^{99m}Tc-MDP bone scintiscans are expected, the availability of merged functional and anatomic information provided by PET/CT and, in the near-future, PET/MR imaging may yield new applications for the widespread use of ^{18}F NaF in clinical practice.

SUMMARY

^{18}F NaF PET/CT is sensitive and specific for the detection of malignant skeletal lesions. It accurately differentiates malignant from benign bone lesions. The higher-quality imaging, increased clinical accuracy, greater convenience to the patient and referring physician, and more efficient use of nuclear medicine resources all indicate the need to reconsider the use of ^{18}F NaF PET for imaging malignant diseases of the skeleton. However, research over a wide area remains to be conducted regarding the use of ^{18}F NaF in malignant bone disease. In addition, future clinical trials required for the validation of preliminary reports on ^{18}F NaF imaging of the skeleton are very likely to be conducted using technologies that are still experimental, such as the combined PET/MR imaging whole-body scanners.

REFERENCES

1. Czernin J, Satyamurthy N, Schiepers C. Molecular mechanisms of bone ^{18}F-NaF deposition. J Nucl Med 2010;51(12):1826–9.
2. Grant FD, Fahey FH, Packard AB, et al. Skeletal PET with ^{18}F-fluoride: applying new technology to an old tracer. J Nucl Med 2008;49(1):68–78.
3. Blau M, Ganatra R, Bender MA. 18 F-fluoride for bone imaging. Semin Nucl Med 1972;2(1):31–7.
4. Bridges RL, Wiley CR, Christian JC, et al. An introduction to Na^{18}F bone scintigraphy: basic principles, advanced imaging concepts, and case examples. J Nucl Med Technol 2007;35(2):64–76.
5. Cook GJ. PET and PET/CT imaging of skeletal metastases. Cancer Imaging 2010;10:1–8.
6. AMI. Academy of Molecular Imaging. 2009. Available at: http://www.ami-imaging.org/index.php?option=com_content&task=view&id=175&Itemid=136. Accessed February 12, 2012.
7. NOPR. National Oncologic PET Registry. 2012. Available at: http://www.cancerpetregistry.org/what.htm. Accessed February 13, 2012.
8. Savelli G, Maffioli L, Maccauro M, et al. Bone scintigraphy and the added value of SPECT (single photon emission tomography) in detecting skeletal lesions. Q J Nucl Med 2001;45(1):27–37.
9. Even-Sapir E. Imaging of malignant bone involvement by morphologic, scintigraphic, and hybrid modalities. J Nucl Med 2005;46(8):1356–67.
10. Even-Sapir E, Metser U, Mishani E, et al. The detection of bone metastases in patients with high-risk prostate cancer: ^{99m}Tc-MDP Planar bone scintigraphy, single- and multi-field-of-view SPECT, ^{18}F-fluoride PET, and ^{18}F-fluoride PET/CT. J Nucl Med 2006;47(2):287–97.
11. Krüger S, Buck A, Mottaghy F, et al. Detection of bone metastases in patients with lung cancer: ^{99m}Tc-MDP planar bone scintigraphy, ^{18}F-fluoride PET or ^{18}F-FDG PET/CT. Eur J Nucl Med Mol Imaging 2009;36(11):1807–12.
12. Schirrmeister H, Guhlmann A, Elsner K, et al. Sensitivity in detecting osseous lesions depends on anatomic localization: planar bone scintigraphy versus ^{18}F PET. J Nucl Med 1999;40(10):1623–9.
13. Iagaru A, Mittra E, Dick D, et al. Prospective evaluation of (99m)Tc MDP scintigraphy, (18)F NaF PET/CT, and (18)F FDG PET/CT for detection of skeletal metastases. Mol Imaging Biol 2012;14(2):252–9.
14. Jemal A, Siegel R, Xu J, et al. Cancer statistics, 2010. CA Cancer J Clin 2010;60(5):277–300.
15. Im H, Kim T, Min H, et al. Prediction of tumour necrosis fractions using metabolic and volumetric ^{18}F-FDG PET/CT indices, after one course and at the completion of neoadjuvant chemotherapy, in children and young adults with osteosarcoma. Eur J Nucl Med Mol Imaging 2012;39(1):39–49.
16. Siegel R, Naishadham D, Jemal A. Cancer statistics, 2012. CA Cancer J Clin 2012;62(1):10–29.
17. Janeway K, Barkauskas D, Krailo M, et al. Outcome for adolescent and young adult patients with osteosarcoma: a report from the Children's Oncology Group. Cancer 2012. [Epub ahead of print].
18. D'Adamo D. Appraising the current role of chemotherapy for the treatment of sarcoma. Semin Oncol 2011;38(Suppl 3):S19–29.
19. Heare T, Hensley M, Dell'Orfano S. Bone tumors: osteosarcoma and Ewing's sarcoma. Curr Opin Pediatr 2009;21(3):365–72.
20. Bajpai J, Sreenivas V, Sharma M, et al. Prediction of chemotherapy response by PET-CT in osteosarcoma: correlation with histologic necrosis. J Pediatr Hematol Oncol 2011;33(7):e271–8.
21. Kim D, Kim S, Lee H, et al. Assessment of chemotherapy response using FDG-PET in pediatric bone tumors: a single institution experience. Cancer Res Treat 2011;43(3):170–5.

22. Iagaru A, Masamed R, Chawla S, et al. F-18 FDG PET and PET/CT evaluation of response to chemotherapy in bone and soft tissue sarcomas. Clin Nucl Med 2008;33(1):8–13.

23. Iagaru A, Quon A, McDougall IR, et al. F-18 FDG PET/CT evaluation of osseous and soft tissue sarcomas. Clin Nucl Med 2006;31(12):754–60.

24. Hoh CK, Hawkins RA, Dahlbom M, et al. Whole body skeletal imaging with [18F]fluoride ion and PET. J Comput Assist Tomogr 1993;17(1):34–41.

25. Tse N, Hoh C, Hawkins R, et al. Positron emission tomography diagnosis of pulmonary metastases in osteogenic sarcoma. Am J Clin Oncol 1994;17(1):22–5.

26. Eary JF, Conrad EU. Imaging in sarcoma. J Nucl Med 2011;52(12):1903–13.

27. Franzius C, Daldrup Link HE, Sciuk J, et al. FDG-PET for detection of pulmonary metastases from malignant primary bone tumors: comparison with spiral CT. Ann Oncol 2001;12(4):479–86.

28. Kaira K, Okumura T, Ohde Y, et al. Correlation between 18F-FDG Uptake on PET and molecular biology in metastatic pulmonary tumors. J Nucl Med 2011;52(5):705–11.

29. Iagaru A, Chawla S, Menendez L, et al. 18F-FDG PET and PET/CT for detection of pulmonary metastases from musculoskeletal sarcomas. Nucl Med Commun 2006;27(10):795–802.

30. Bernstein M, Kovar H, Paulussen M, et al. Ewing's sarcoma family of tumors: current management. Oncologist 2006;11(5):503–19.

31. Walter F, Federman N, Apichairuk W, et al. 18F-fluorodeoxyglucose uptake of bone and soft tissue sarcomas in pediatric patients. Pediatr Hematol Oncol 2011;28(7):579–87.

32. Gaston L, Di Bella C, Slavin J, et al. 18F-FDG PET response to neoadjuvant chemotherapy for Ewing sarcoma and osteosarcoma are different. Skeletal Radiol 2011;40(8):1007–15.

33. Angtuaco EJ, Fassas AB, Walker R, et al. Multiple myeloma: clinical review and diagnostic imaging1. Radiology 2004;231(1):11–23.

34. Winterbottom AP, Shaw AS. Imaging patients with myeloma. Clin Radiol 2009;64(1):1–11.

35. Collins C. Multiple myeloma. Cancer Imaging 2004; 4(Spec No A):S47–53.

36. Ludwig H, Kumpan W, Sinzinger H. Radiography and bone scintigraphy in multiple myeloma: a comparative analysis. Br J Radiol 1982;55(651): 173–81.

37. Kurdziel K, Lindenberg L, Mena E, et al. Temporal characterization of F-18 NaF PET/CT uptake. J Nucl Med Meeting Abstracts 2011;52(1):459.

38. Even-Sapir E, Metser U, Flusser G, et al. Assessment of malignant skeletal disease: initial experience with 18F-fluoride PET/CT and comparison between 18F-fluoride PET and 18F-fluoride PET/CT. J Nucl Med 2004;45(2):272–8.

39. Picchio M, Messa C, Landoni C, et al. Value of [11C] choline-positron emission tomography for re-staging prostate cancer: a comparison with [18F]fluorodeoxyglucose-positron emission tomography. J Urol 2003;169(4):1337–40.

40. Jadvar H, Desai B, Conti P, et al. Preliminary evaluation of 18F-NaF and 18F-FDG PET/CT in detection of metastatic disease in men with PSA relapse after treatment for localized primary prostate cancer. J Nucl Med Meeting Abstracts 2011;52(1):1916.

41. Picchio M, Giovannini E, Messa C. The role of PET/computed tomography scan in the management of prostate cancer. Curr Opin Urol 2011; 21(3):230–6.

42. Langsteger W, Balogova S, Huchet V, et al. Fluorocholine (18F) and sodium fluoride (18F) PET/CT in the detection of prostate cancer: prospective comparison of diagnostic performance determined by masked reading. Q J Nucl Med Mol Imaging 2011;55(4):448–57.

43. Cook G, Parker C, Chua S, et al. 18F-fluoride PET: changes in uptake as a method to assess response in bone metastases from castrate-resistant prostate cancer patients treated with 223Ra-chloride (Alpharadin). EJNMMI Res 2011;1(1):4.

44. Coleman RE, Seaman JJ. The role of zoledronic acid in cancer: clinical studies in the treatment and prevention of bone metastases. Semin Oncol 2001; 28(2 Suppl 6):11–6.

45. Yamashita K, Koyama H, Inaji H. Prognostic significance of bone metastasis from breast cancer. Clin Orthop Relat Res 1995;(312):89–94.

46. Petrn-Mallmin M, Andrasson I, Ljunggren O, et al. Skeletal metastases from breast cancer: uptake of 18F-fluoride measured with positron emission tomography in correlation with CT. Skeletal Radiol 1998; 27(2):72–6.

47. Doot RK, Muzi M, Peterson LM, et al. Kinetic analysis of 18F-Fluoride PET images of breast cancer bone metastases. J Nucl Med 2010;51(4):521–7.

48. Tritz DB, Doll DC, Ringenberg QS, et al. Bone marrow involvement in small cell lung cancer. Clinical significance and correlation with routine laboratory variables. Cancer 1989;63(4):763–6.

49. Bezwoda WR, Lewis D, Livini N. Bone marrow involvement in anaplastic small cell lung cancer. Diagnosis, hematologic features, and prognostic implications. Cancer 1986;58(8):1762–5.

50. Trillet V, Revel D, Combaret V, et al. Bone marrow metastases in small cell lung cancer: detection with magnetic resonance imaging and monoclonal antibodies. Br J Cancer 1989;60(1):83–8.

51. Schirrmeister H, Glatting G, Hetzel J Jr, et al. Prospective evaluation of the clinical value of planar bone scans, SPECT, and 18F-Labeled NaF PET in newly diagnosed lung cancer. J Nucl Med 2001; 42(12):1800–4.

52. Hetzel M, Arslandemir C, Knig HH, et al. F-18 NaF PET for detection of bone metastases in lung cancer: accuracy, cost-effectiveness, and impact on patient management. J Bone Miner Res 2003;18(12):2206–14.

53. Iagaru A, Mittra E, Yaghoubi SS, et al. Novel strategy for a cocktail ^{18}F-fluoride and ^{18}F-FDG PET/CT scan for evaluation of malignancy: results of the pilot-phase study. J Nucl Med 2009;50(4):501–5.

54. Lin F, Rao J, Mittra E, et al. Prospective comparison of combined (18)F-FDG and (18)F-NaF PET/CT vs. (18)F-FDG PET/CT imaging for detection of malignancy. Eur J Nucl Med Mol Imaging 2012;39(2):262–70.

55. Iagaru A, Mittra E, Sathekge M, et al. Combined ^{18}F-NaF and ^{18}F FDG PET/CT: initial results of a multicenter trial. J Nucl Med Meeting Abstracts 2011; 52(1):34.

Quantitative PET Imaging Using ^{18}F Sodium Fluoride in the Assessment of Metabolic Bone Diseases and the Monitoring of Their Response to Therapy

Glen M. Blake, PhD[a],*, Musib Siddique, PhD[a], Michelle L. Frost, PhD[a],
Amelia E.B. Moore, PhD[a], Ignac Fogelman, MD[b]

KEYWORDS

- Osteoporosis • Paget's disease • Regional bone turnover • Positron emission tomography
- ^{18}F sodium fluoride • Quantitative imaging • Bone plasma clearance • Standardized uptake value

KEY POINTS

- Bone turnover markers have an important role in research studying the effect of new treatments for osteoporosis on bone metabolism.
- Bone turnover markers respond to the integrated effects of treatment across the entire skeleton.
- Positron emission tomography with ^{18}F-sodium fluoride (^{18}F NaF PET) provides a novel tool for studying bone metabolism that can measure the effects of treatment at specific sites, such as the spine and hip.
- Dynamic ^{18}F NaF PET imaging can be used to measure the effective bone plasma flow (from which bone blood flow can be estimated) and the ^{18}F NaF plasma clearance to bone mineral at sites within the field of view of the PET scanner.
- Bone plasma clearance may also be estimated from a series of static scans performed at multiple sites throughout the skeleton with a single injection of ^{18}F NaF, provided that venous blood samples are taken to estimate the input function.
- Standardized uptake values in bone may also be measured but, unlike bone plasma clearance, they are influenced by changes occurring elsewhere in the skeleton away from the measurement site.
- ^{18}F NaF PET studies have confirmed that osteoporosis treatments can have different effects at different sites in the skeleton.
- ^{18}F NaF PET is a useful research tool for future studies.

MEASUREMENTS OF BONE TURNOVER

Over the past 20 years, a series of increasingly potent new treatments have been licensed for the prevention of osteoporotic fractures (**Table 1**).[1–8] The most commonly used class of drugs used to treat osteoporosis are the bisphosphonate (BP), which are also widely used for the treatment of Paget's disease of bone.[9] Many of the therapies listed in **Table 1** have a profound effect on bone remodeling, and studies of bone turnover play an important role in research studies to evaluate their

[a] Osteoporosis Unit, King's College London, King's Health Partners, Guy's Hospital, London SE1 9RT, UK;
[b] Department of Nuclear Medicine, King's College London, King's Health Partners, Guy's Hospital, London SE1 9RT, UK
* Corresponding author. Osteoporosis Research Unit, 1st Floor, Tower Wing, Guy's Hospital, London SE1 9RT, UK.
E-mail address: glen.blake@kcl.ac.uk

PET Clin 7 (2012) 275–291
doi:10.1016/j.cpet.2012.04.001

Table 1
Treatments for osteoporosis and other metabolic bone diseases

Mode of Action	Class of Drug	Name (Commercial Name)
Antiresorptive	Bisphosphonates	Etidronate (Didronel PMO)
		Alendronic acid (Fosamax)
		Risedronate (Actonel)
		Ibandronic acid (Bonviva)
		Zoledronic acid (Aclasta)
	Selective estrogen receptor modulator	Raloxifene (Evista)
	Human monoclonal antibody	Denosumab (Prolia)
Anabolic	Recombinant human parathyroid hormone	Teriparatide (Forsteo)

effect on bone quality.[10–14] Bone remodeling refers to the cycle of resorption and replacement of bone tissue by osteoclasts and osteoblasts, respectively.[15] The assessment of bone turnover is important for monitoring patients with osteoporosis and Paget's disease, and is used to quantify response to treatment and evaluate drug effectiveness in clinical trials.[16,17]

The gold standard for the assessment of bone remodeling is bone biopsy with double tetracycline labelling.[11–14] This technique is, however, complex, costly, and invasive, and is restricted to a single site, the iliac crest. A more commonly used and practical method is the measurement of biochemical markers of bone resorption and bone formation in serum and urine, which have the advantage that a large and rapid response is seen in patients commencing treatment for osteoporosis with the therapies listed in **Table 1**.[16,17] However, because biochemical markers respond to the global changes occurring across the whole skeleton, they cannot provide insight into the changes that occur at specific sites of interest, such as investigating differences between trabecular and cortical

bone, or monitoring the response to treatment at sites of clinically important osteoporotic fractures, such as the hip and spine.

Radionuclide imaging using positron emission tomography (PET) with the short half-life bone-seeking tracer fluorine-18–labeled sodium fluoride (^{18}F NaF) ($T_{1/2}$ = 110 minutes) or gamma camera studies using the nuclear medicine bone scan agent technetium-99m-methylene diphosphonate (^{99m}Tc-MDP) ($T_{1/2}$ = 6.0 hours) provide a unique way of investigating regional bone metabolism that complements bone biopsy and biochemical markers as a tool for research studies.[18,19] Radionuclide tracers bind to newly mineralizing bone and serve as markers of bone blood flow and osteoblastic activity.[20] The mechanism of uptake is the deposition of ^{18}F NaF or ^{99m}Tc-MDP on the surface of newly forming hydroxyapatite crystals at sites of bone formation, and hence the aspect of bone turnover being measured is related to the recent level of osteoblastic activity.[21,22] The advantage of imaging techniques such as ^{18}F NaF PET and ^{99m}Tc-MDP gamma camera scans is their flexibility in that they can be used to study not only the whole skeleton but also any chosen region of interest (ROI).

Blau and colleagues[23] were the first to recognize ^{18}F NaF as an excellent tracer for skeletal imaging with a high affinity for bone that leads to a large tissue to background ratio and hence good-quality images. As PET scanners have become more widely available in the past 20 years, ^{18}F NaF has assumed an increasingly important role in nuclear medicine bone imaging.[24,25] The fluoride ion is believed to exchange with the hydroxyl groups in hydroxyapatite crystals on the surface of the bone matrix to form fluoroapatite[25,26]:

$$Ca_5(PO_4)_3OH + F^- \rightarrow Ca_5(PO_4)_3F + OH^-$$

As with other bone-seeking tracers, uptake of ^{18}F NaF is concentrated preferentially at sites of newly mineralizing bone.[27–31] Although the rate-limiting step controlling uptake is bone blood flow,[26] uptake is also influenced by changes in osteoblastic activity.[32,33]

An important advantage of ^{18}F NaF compared with ^{99m}Tc-MDP for quantitative studies of bone tracer kinetics is the absence of binding to plasma proteins,[34] and therefore studies to measure plasma clearance are not complicated by the need to measure protein binding. The good spatial resolution of PET images compared with the gamma camera and the fact that PET provides three-dimensional (3D) tomographic images rather than two-dimensional (2D) planar images are additional advantages of ^{18}F NaF PET over ^{99m}Tc-MDP gamma camera studies.[19,33] Tomographic images are preferable to planar ones because they provide bone uptake measurements and bone time-activity curves (TACs) free of any contribution from overlying soft tissue. These and other advantages of ^{18}F NaF for quantitative imaging of bone tracer kinetics are summarized in **Box 1**.

QUANTITATIVE PET IMAGING USING ^{18}F NAF
The Hawkins Method

Quantitative ^{18}F NaF PET studies are often performed using the dynamic scan method first described by Hawkins and colleagues.[18] Quantitative ^{18}F NaF PET was the first radionuclide imaging technique to measure bone plasma clearance rather than bone uptake, and the method has since been widely adopted by other researchers.[32,33,35–37] The typical value of the ^{18}F NaF plasma clearance to bone mineral in the lumbar spine is 0.03 mL min^{-1} mL^{-1} (eg, the amount of tracer taken up in 1 mL of bone tissue in 1 minute is the same as that transported in 0.03 mL of plasma).

With the Hawkins method, the patient receives a bolus injection of ^{18}F NaF in a 10-mL saline solution while a 60-minute dynamic PET scan simultaneously images the chosen site in the skeleton. A set of protocols for image acquisition and reconstruction are summarized in **Box 2**. The bone ROIs are restricted to the 15-cm section of the human body that can be included in the field of view of the PET scanner, such as the lumbar spine (L1–L4) or the hip (**Fig. 1**). To measure bone plasma clearance, the arterial input function (IF) must also be found, which can be achieved either through direct monitoring using an arterial blood line,[18,35–37] using an image-derived input function from an ROI placed over the abdominal aorta,[36] or using a population-derived curve calibrated against venous blood samples obtained 30 to 60 minutes after injection.[33]

The object of the dynamic PET scan is to obtain the TACs for the concentration of ^{18}F NaF in the bone ROI and arterial blood during the first 60

Box 2
Protocols for PET image acquisition and reconstruction

60-minute dynamic study on PET/CT scanner

Scan mode: 2D

Frame times: twenty-four 5-second, four 30-second, and fourteen 240-second frames

Patient preparation: patient should be well hydrated and comfortable on scan table

CT scout scan: 10 mA at 120 kV$_p$

Patient positioning:

    Spine: L1–L4, including bottom of T12 and top of L5

    Hip: 1 cm above acetabulum to mid–femoral shaft

Injected activity: 90 MBq (lumbar spine) or 180 MBq (hip) ^{18}F NaF in 10 mL saline

Injection protocol

    T0: start dynamic scan

    T0 + 10 seconds: start injection of ^{18}F NaF

    T0 + 20 seconds: finish injection; follow with 10 mL saline flush

    T0 + 30 seconds: finish saline flush

Blood sampling (for semi-population arterial input function):

    Venous blood samples (1.5 mL) from opposite arm to injection at 30, 40, 50, and 60 minutes

Reconstruction parameters:

    Matrix size: 128 × 128

    Reconstruction: filtered back projection

    Attenuation correction: from CT image

    Transaxial filter: Hanning 6.3 mm

    Randoms correction: correction from singles

    Deadtime correction: yes

    Scatter correction: yes

Box 1
Advantages of ^{18}F NaF as a bone tracer

- High and rapid bone uptake
- Rapid clearance from blood
- High bone to soft tissue background by 45 to 60 minutes
- No protein binding
- Superior image quality of ^{18}F NaF PET
- Widespread availability of PET scanners

---

minutes after the bolus injection (**Fig. 2**). Both curves are corrected for radioactive decay of ^{18}F back to the time of injection. These curves are then analyzed using the compartmental model (the Hawkins model) shown in **Fig. 3** to find the effective bone plasma flow to bone tissue (K_1) and the plasma clearance to the bone mineral compartment (K_i).[18] In the Hawkins model, the rate constant K_1 describes the clearance of ^{18}F-NaF from plasma to the unbound bone pool, k_2 the reverse transport from the unbound bone

A

B

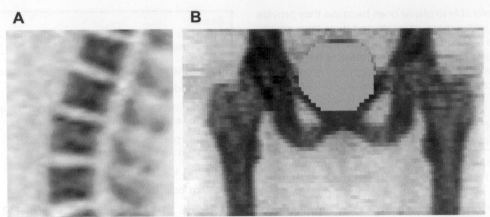

Fig. 1. ^{18}F NaF PET images showing (*A*) a sagittal image of the lumbar spine (L1–L4) and (*B*) a coronal image of the proximal femur. Both images are 2D projection views of the complete 3D PET scan data, and both are restricted to the 15-cm axial field of view of the PET scanner. In the femur image, ^{18}F NaF activity collecting in the urinary bladder during the 1-hour dynamic scan has been masked to give a clearer view of the uptake in bone. (*From Blake GM, Frost ML, Moore AE, et al. The assessment of regional skeletal metabolism: studies of osteoporosis treatments using quantitative radionuclide imaging. J Clin Densitom 2011;14:263–71; with permission from the International Society for Clinical Densitometry.*)

pool back to plasma, k_3 the forward transport from the unbound bone pool to bone mineral, and k_4 the reverse flow. Bone blood flow can be estimated from K_1 knowing the packed cell volume and the first pass extraction of ^{18}F NaF, which is often assumed to be 100%.[38,39] The parameter K_i representing the plasma clearance of ^{18}F NaF to bone mineral is calculated using Equation 1[18]:

$$K_i = K_1 \times k_3/(k_2 + k_3) \text{ mL min}^{-1} \text{ mL}^{-1} \quad (1)$$

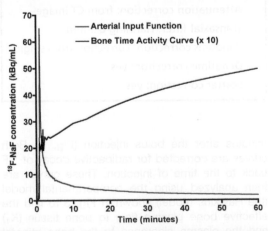

Fig. 2. A representative study showing the arterial input function measured by direct blood sampling and corresponding bone TAC for a ^{18}F NaF dynamic PET scan of the lumbar spine. Both curves have been corrected for radioactive decay.

In Equation 1, the ratio $k_3/(k_2 + k_3)$ represents the fraction of tracer initially cleared to bone tissue that binds to bone mineral and takes values between 0 and 1.0. The use of K_i to study bone formation was validated in two reports that found correlations with histomorphometric indices of bone formation and mineral apposition rate.[21,22] Alternative methods to the Hawkins model for analyzing the bone TAC and IF curves to evaluate K_1 and K_i include deconvolution and spectral analysis.[40] A fourth method described later, the Patlak plot, provides a simple graphical method of evaluating K_i but cannot be used to find K_1.[40]

The results of the Hawkins model fit to the bone ROI time-activity and arterial plasma input curves are shown in **Fig. 4.** The fit to the model is obtained through varying the values of the four parameters in **Fig. 3** until the predicted TAC for the bone ROI gives the closest fit to the measured curve. The

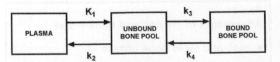

Fig. 3. The Hawkins compartmental model used for the analysis of ^{18}F NaF PET dynamic bone scans.[18] The rate constant K_1 describes the effective bone plasma flow to the unbound bone pool, k_2 the reverse transport of tracer from the unbound bone pool back to plasma, k_3 the forward transport from the unbound bone pool to bone mineral, and k_4 the reverse flow.

value of K_i is then calculated using Equation 1. The model also allows the fractional volume of the bone ROI occupied by blood to be fitted as a free parameter, which can improve the fit to the data in the first 30 seconds after the injection of tracer. **Fig. 4** shows time plots of the amount of tracer in each of the three compartments in **Fig. 3** and the resulting fit of the summed curves to the bone ROI TAC. Images and curves should always be closely scrutinized before results of model fits are accepted. Dynamic scans should be checked for possible patient movement before undertaking quantitative analysis. Some points for evaluating curve fits are discussed in **Fig. 5**.

The Patlak Plot Method

When the rate constant k_4 for the backflow of tracer from the bone mineral compartment to the unbound bone pool is negligibly small ($1/k_4$ >>60 minutes), the Patlak plot method provides a computationally simple method of estimating K_i from the slope of a straight-line graph (**Fig. 6A**).[18] The method is based on the assumption that the total amount of tracer in the bone ROI is given by Equation 2[41]:

$$C_{tissue}(T) = K_i \int_0^T C_{plasma}(t)dt + V_0 C_{plasma}(T) \quad (2)$$

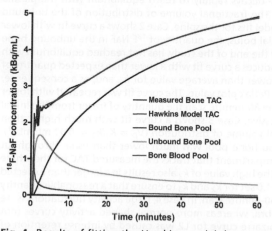

Fig. 4. Results of fitting the Hawkins model shown to the bone TAC and arterial plasma input function shown in **Fig. 2**. In addition to the four parameters K_1, k_2, k_3 and k_4, the model also fits the fractional volume of blood within the bone ROI, F_{BV}. The plasma clearance to bone mineral K_i is calculated using Equation 1. The figure shows time activity plots of the amount of tracer in each of the three compartments shown in **Fig. 3** and the resulting fit of the summed curves to the measured bone TAC.

where t is time, $C_{tissue}(T)$ is the total amount of tracer in the bone ROI at time T after injection, $C_{plasma}(T)$ is the concentration of tracer in plasma, K_i is the bone plasma clearance, and V_0 is the volume of distribution of tracer in the bone ROI. The first term on the right-hand-side of Equation 2 represents the amount of tracer in the bone mineral compartment in **Fig. 3**, and the second term the amount of the tracer in the unbound bone pool. By dividing both sides of Equation 2 by $C_{plasma}(T)$ a straight-line relationship is obtained with slope K_i and intercept V_0 (see **Fig. 6A**). To allow for equilibration between tracer in plasma and the unbound bone pool, the values of K_i and V_0 are determined through fitting the dynamic scan data from 10 to 60 minutes after injection.[41]

For [18]F NaF the assumption that k_4 is negligibly small is not strictly valid ($1/k_4$ ~ 100 minutes). As a consequence, the final (50–60 minute) points of the Patlak plot can deviate slightly from the straight line, and Patlak K_i measurements tend to underestimate the Hawkins model results by around 25% on average (see **Fig. 6B**).[40] Comparison of the goodness of fit to the bone TAC between the Hawkins model with $k_4 = 0$ and the model with k_4 fitted as a free parameter using the Akaike information criterion[42] show that the latter generally provides a statistically significantly better fit to the data.[40] Hence, the Patlak method clearly gives a less accurate estimate of K_i than the Hawkins model because it ignores k_4. However, for the same reason, the Patlak method provides values of K_i with better precision than the Hawkins model because it eliminates the effect of the random measurement errors in k_2, k_3, and k_4 on values of K_i.[40] As discussed later, the better precision of the Patlak analysis makes it the preferred method for evaluating K_i in longitudinal studies.[40] However, the method cannot be used to evaluate K_1.

Standardized Uptake Values

A simpler method of quantifying PET studies that avoids the need to find the input function is to measure standardized uptake values (SUVs) through normalizing the mean [18]F NaF concentration in the bone region of interest for injected activity and body weight: SUV$_{mean}$ = mean kBq/mL × body weight (kg)/injected activity (MBq).[43] In PET studies that image malignant disease, maximum or peak values of SUV are commonly evaluated, and this practice can be justified based on the frequent lack of homogeneity of tracer uptake seen in tumors.[44] However, in osteoporosis and other types of diffuse metabolic bone disease, the [18]F NaF uptake in bone tissue such as the vertebral body or the femoral shaft is uniform,

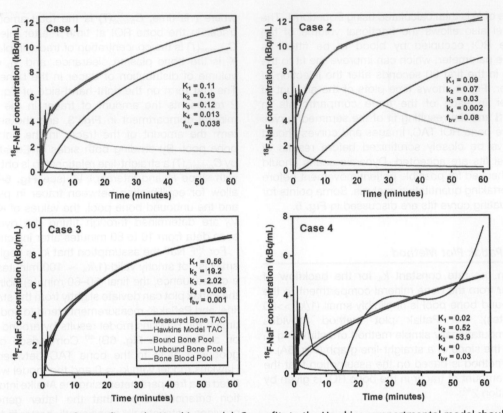

Fig. 5. Evaluation of curve fits to the Hawkins model. Curve fits to the Hawkins compartmental model should not be blindly accepted, but the quality of the curve fits should be evaluated visually for any technical problems. Suitable starting conditions for the Hawkins model fit to the bone TAC are: $K_1 = 0.1$; $k_2 = 0.2$; $k_3 = 0.1$; $k_4 = 0.01$; and F_{BV} (fractional blood volume) = 0.03. Case 1 shows an ideal curve fit with the final best-fit parameters not far from the starting conditions. The fractional blood volume is not excessive, the value of k_4 is reasonable, and, after the initial bolus, the quantity of ^{18}F NaF in the unbound bone pool decays rapidly to reach equilibrium with the plasma compartment well before the end of the 60-minute scan. The fractional volume of distribution of the unbound bone pool ($V_D = K_1/k_2 \approx 0.5$ mL mL^{-1}) is typical of many model fits for the spine. Case 2 shows a curve fit with lower than average values of k_2 and k_3. As a result, after the initial bolus, the quantity of ^{18}F NaF in the unbound bone pool remains high throughout the 60-minute scan, and, by the end of the study, has not reached equilibrium with the plasma compartment. As a consequence, the model produces a curve fit with a lower than expected quantity of tracer in the bone mineral compartment at 60 minutes, a lower than average value for k_4, and, as a consequence, a lower than expected value of K_i that was smaller than the Patlak plot value. The curve fit was repeated with lower limits of 0.1 set for k_2 and k_3 to ensure that at the end of the 60-minute scan the quantity of tracer from the initial bolus remaining in the unbound bone pool was not excessive. Case 3 shows a curve fit with much higher than average values of k_2 and k_3 and a much smaller that usual volume of distribution ($V_D = K_1/k_2 \approx 0.03$ mL mL^{-1}). As a consequence, the amount of ^{18}F NaF in the unbound bone pool was much lower than usual throughout the 60-minute scan, resulting in a TAC for bone mineral compartment that tracks the measured TAC for the whole bone ROI and consequently overestimates the value of K_i. The high value of k_2 also results in a larger than expected value of K_1. The curve fit was repeated with upper limits of 1.0 set for k_2 and k_3 to ensure that a reasonable quantity of tracer exists in the unbound bone pool throughout the 60-minute scan. In Case 4, large activity fluctuations were seen in the measured bone TAC for the L2 lumbar vertebra, whereas more normal-shaped activity curves (not shown) were seen for the L1, L3, and L4 vertebrae. The bizarre curve for L2 was caused by intense retention of ^{18}F NaF tracer in the adjacent renal calyces, the proximity of which caused streaking artifacts in PET images reconstructed using filtered back projection (see **Fig. 14**). The curve fit for the subject was repeated after averaging the bone TACs for L1, L3, and L4.

and so the mean SUV within the bone ROI is a more appropriate index than the maximum value.

One disadvantage of the Hawkins method is that with a single injection of ^{18}F NaF, only a single

60-minute dynamic scan at one chosen site in the skeleton can be performed. Therefore, the measurements are restricted to the 15-cm field of view of the PET scanner (see **Fig. 1**). In contrast,

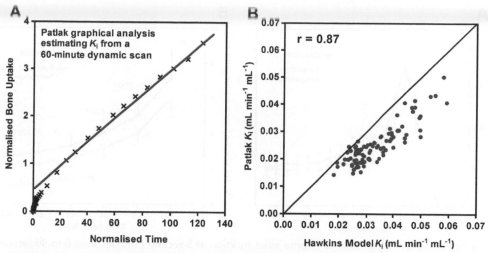

Fig. 6. (A) Patlak plot of ^{18}F NaF PET study data obtained during a 60-minute dynamic scan. The graph is a plot of normalized uptake ($C_{tissue}(T)/C_{plasma}(T)$) against normalized time ($\int_0^T C_{plasma}(t)dt/C_{plasma}(T)$) (see Equation 2). Fluoride plasma clearance to bone mineral (K_i) is found from the slope of the straight-line fit to the 10- to 60-minute data points. The intercept on the vertical axis gives the volume of distribution. (B) Scatter plot for values of lumbar spine K_i determined using the Patlak plot method against results when the same dynamic scans were analyzed using the Hawkins model. Patlak plot K_i values are systematically lower than the Hawkins model values by approximately 25% because they ignore the effect of the backflow of tracer out of bone (k_4). The scatter in the results is caused by the random errors in fitting k_2, k_3, and k_4 to the bone TAC.

SUV measurements have the advantage that they require only a short (~5 minutes) static scan at the measurement site compared with the 60-minute scan required by the Hawkins method. Hence, with a series of static scans starting 30 to 40 minutes after injection, SUVs can be measured over most of the skeleton during a period when the bone TAC is only slowly changing (see **Fig. 2**). Recently, Siddique and colleagues[41] described how, with the addition of two to four venous measurements of ^{18}F NaF plasma concentration obtained 30 to 60 minutes after injection, reliable estimates of Patlak K_i values can be obtained from static ^{18}F NaF PET scans. Therefore, both K_i and SUV values can now be estimated across most of the skeleton from a series of short static scans obtained after a single injection of tracer. This method is described in greater detail later.

Bone Plasma Clearance or SUV?

A key question is whether SUV measurements of bone uptake provide equivalent information to plasma clearance about changes in bone metabolism, or whether the additional complexity of taking blood samples to find the input function results in any demonstrable improvement in the reliability of the PET scan findings.[45] If the effect of bone diseases or treatments on whole-body ^{18}F NaF kinetics are not large enough to significantly alter the input function, then there is little point in taking

blood, because measurements of SUV and K_i will yield similar information. Although this is probably true in most circumstances, some of the treatments listed in **Table 1** have such a potent effect on bone turnover, either in the whole skeleton or localized areas of Pagetic bone, that the whole-body kinetics of ^{18}F NaF, including the plasma TAC after the bolus peak, is significantly altered (**Fig. 7**).[45] Similarly, for some cases of Paget's disease and in some patients with extensive bone metastases (described as *superscans*), the uptake in bone lesions is so elevated that the presence of the disease alters the arterial input function of bone-seeking tracers from the curves typically seen in healthy subjects.[46,47]

The limitation of SUVs or any other type of bone uptake measurement is that only a finite amount of tracer is available for sharing out between competing sites (normal bone, bony lesions, or the kidneys).[48] Any large change in plasma clearance at one site can therefore alter the amount of tracer available for uptake at other sites. Thus, SUVs reflect not only changes in bone tracer kinetics at the measurement site but also, through their effect on the input function, the changes occurring in other areas of the skeleton. In contrast, plasma clearance measurements quantify the local uptake of tracer in terms of its availability in the circulation. They are therefore a more specific measurement of the true changes in bone tracer kinetics occurring at the measurement site. This

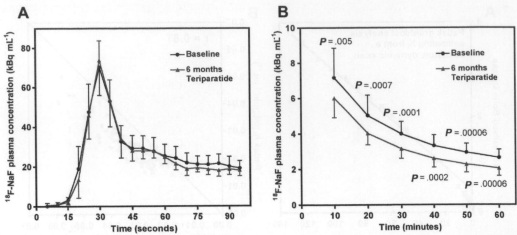

Fig. 7. (A) Plot of mean ^{18}F NaF arterial plasma input function at 5-second intervals from 0 to 90 seconds after start of PET scan image acquisition. The two curves are for the scans acquired at baseline and after 6 months of treatment with teriparatide.[33] The data show the image-derived input functions obtained at the abdominal aorta. (B) Plot of mean ^{18}F NaF venous plasma activity concentrations at 10, 20, 30, 40, 50, and 60 minutes after injection before and after teriparatide treatment from the study shown in (A). ^{18}F NaF activity was corrected for radioactive decay.

effect is illustrated in the example shown in **Fig. 8** taken from a study of the effect of teriparatide treatment on ^{18}F NaF kinetics in the spine.[45] Although 6 months of treatment with teriparatide resulted in a 24% increase in bone plasma clearance, the effects across the whole skeleton were sufficiently

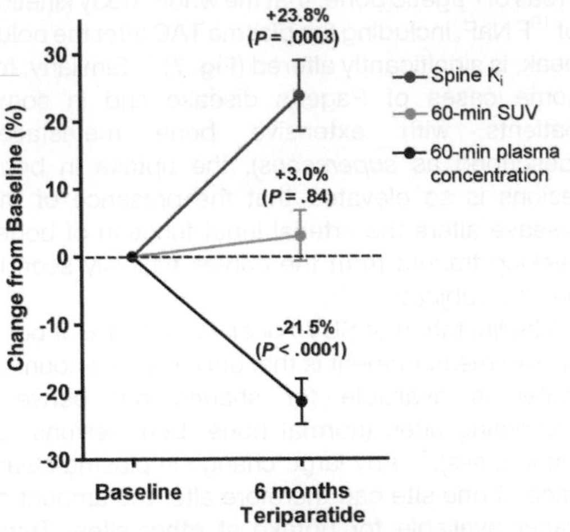

Fig. 8. Plot showing the mean changes in (1) ^{18}F NaF lumbar spine plasma clearance (K_i) measured using the Hawkins model, (2) lumbar spine SUV (52- to 60-minute values), and (3) 60-minute ^{18}F NaF venous plasma activity concentration, all after 6 months of treatment with teriparatide. (*Data from* Blake GM, Siddique M, Frost ML, et al. Radionuclide studies of bone metabolism: do bone uptake and bone plasma clearance provide equivalent measurements of bone turnover? Bone 2011;49:537–42.)

large to produce a 20% decrease in the plasma concentration TAC (see **Fig. 7**B). Hence the change in SUV at the spine was only 3% and was not statistically significantly different from zero.[45]

Measurements of Bone Blood Flow

Measurements of bone plasma clearance (K_i) require accurate information on the bone TAC and the arterial input function for the full 60-minute dynamic scan (see **Fig. 4**). An approximate value of K_i (based on the assumptions that $k_4 = 0$ and tracer in the unbound bone pool can be ignored) is obtained through dividing the bone activity concentration at 60 minutes by the area under the plasma curve (AUC) from 0 to 60 minutes ($K_i \sim$ bone ROI activity [60 minutes]/AUC [0–60 minutes]). In contrast, measurements of the effective bone plasma flow (K_1) depend on the dynamic scan data obtained during the 30-second interval over the peak of the bolus injection (**Fig. 9**). An approximate value of K_1 (based on the assumptions that no backflow of tracer from the unbound bone pool to plasma is present and that tracer in the blood volume within bone tissue can be ignored) is obtained by dividing the bone activity concentration at 30 seconds after the start of the bolus by the AUC under the bolus peak ($K_1 \sim$ bone ROI activity [30 seconds]/AUC [0–30 seconds]). The typical value of K_1 in the lumbar spine is 0.1 mL min^{-1} mL^{-1}, or approximately three times larger than the typical value of K_i.

Piert and colleagues[39,49] compared ^{18}F NaF PET measurements of K_1 in pigs with equivalent data obtained using the freely diffusible tracer

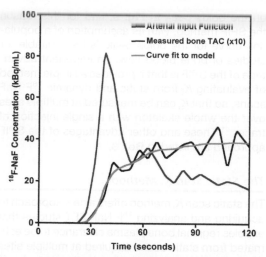

Fig. 9. Results of curve fit to bone TAC and the arterial input function during the first 120 seconds after the start of dynamic PET scan image acquisition. The data were fitted to the Hawkins model (see **Fig. 3**), with $k_3 = 0$ to derive K_1 and k_2.

^{15}O-H$_2$O, a standard technique for measuring regional blood flow in PET studies. The results showed good agreement between the measurements at low flow rates consistent with 100% first pass extraction of ^{18}F NaF, but at normal and elevated flow rates, the ^{18}F NaF K_1 measurements underestimated the results of the ^{15}O-H$_2$O studies (**Fig. 10A**), probably because the first pass extraction of fluoride became diffusion-limited at high

flow rates. The results were consistent with the Renkin-Crone relationship (Equation 3)[50,51]:

$$K_1 = f \cdot E_F = f \cdot [1 - \exp(-PS/f)] \qquad (3)$$

where f is the true flow rate, E_F the unidirectional extraction fraction of ^{18}F NaF, and PS the permeability-surface area product of the capillary bed. After correction for the permeability-surface area product, a linear relationship was obtained (see **Fig. 10B**).

Measurements of the Arterial Input Function

To obtain reliable results for K_1 and K_i, the analysis of ^{18}F NaF PET data requires accurate measurement of the input function. This measurement can be obtained in several ways: (1) continuous arterial sampling using an online blood monitor,[35–37] (2) arterial blood samples obtained at discrete time points postinjection, (3) a population-based IF,[36] or (4) an image-derived input function (IDIF) obtained by placing an ROI over an artery and calibrating the resulting curves against venous blood samples obtained during the later phases (30–60 minutes) of the dynamic scan when venous and arterial ^{18}F concentrations are equal.[36,52–54]

Although continuous arterial blood sampling is the most reliable method, it is invasive and requires the presence of personnel trained in arterial cannulation. The use of a population-based input function is generally considered unsuitable because the adopted blood curve may not be appropriate

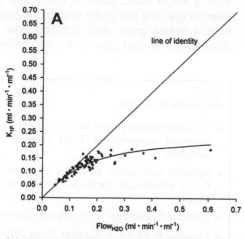

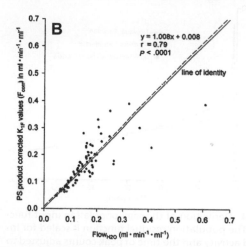

Fig. 10. (A) Plot of effective bone plasma flow (K_1) measured using ^{18}F NaF PET against the corresponding flow measurements made using ^{15}O-H$_2$O in pig vertebrae.[39] The plot shows the trend for ^{18}F NaF PET measurements to underestimate true bone blood flow at higher flow rates. (B) Correction of the relationship shown in (A) using the Rankin-Crone relationship (Equation 3) to correct for the permeability-surface area product. (*From* Piert M, Zittel TT, Machulla HJ, et al. Blood flow measurements with [^{15}O]H$_2$O and [^{18}F]fluoride ion PET in porcine vertebrae. J Bone Miner Res 1998;13:1328–36; with permission from the American Society of Bone and Mineral Research.)

for the individual or population being studied.[36] Image-derived input functions provide a practical alternative, but require correction for the partial volume effect and background spillover.[36,52–54] In practice for [18]F NaF studies of the spine, the proximity of the abdominal aorta to areas of high tracer uptake in the vertebrae and other adjacent features means that the artery is only clearly visualized against the surrounding background during the 30-second period of the bolus peak, making it difficult to reliably estimate the IDIF over the full 60 minutes of the dynamic scan. For this reason, Frost and colleagues developed a semi-population input function (SPIF) that uses venous blood samples obtained 30 to 60 minutes after injection (when arterial and venous blood levels are in equilibrium) to find the terminal exponential of the 0- to 60-minute plasma curve, and adds a population residual curve adjusted for injected activity and the time of peak count rate to represent the bolus and fast exponentials (**Fig. 11**).[33]

Because the terminal exponential accounts for more than 75% of the 0- to 60-minute AUC, and because no evidence shows that even therapies that have a potent effect on bone turnover can alter the bolus peak (see **Fig. 7A**), the effect of variations in the residual curve between individuals on estimations of [18]F NaF plasma clearance is minimal. In contrast, reliable estimates of K_1 require an accurate knowledge of the true input function during the 30-second period centered

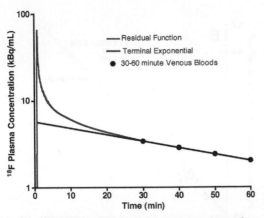

Fig. 11. Derivation of the semi-population input function. The population residual function is scaled for injected activity and the time of peak counts adjusted to agree with a region of interest drawn over the aorta on the PET image data. This curve is added to the terminal exponential fitted to the 30-, 40-, 50-, and 60-minute venous plasma data. The terminal exponential is rolled off using a ramp function at the time of peak counts so as not to affect the early rise of the bolus.

on the bolus peak in **Fig. 9**, and for this reason the SPIF method, with its assumption of a population curve for the bolus peak, is less suitable for studies of bone blood flow. An important advantage of the SPIF is that it provides a simple method of evaluating K_i from static and dynamic [18]F NaF scans, so that K_i can be measured at multiple sites over the whole skeleton with a single injection of tracer.[41] These and other advantages of the SPIF approach are listed in **Box 3**.

The Static Scan K_i Method

The static scan K_i method offers a new approach to acquiring and analyzing [18]F NaF PET studies that enables regional bone plasma clearance to be estimated from static scans acquired at multiple sites in the skeleton after a single injection of tracer.[41] The method requires a small number (two to four) of venous blood samples 30 to 60 minutes after injection to evaluate the terminal exponential component of the SPIF (see **Fig. 11**). On rearranging Equation 2, one obtains Equation 4:

$$K_i = \frac{\left[\dfrac{C_{tissue}(T)}{C_{plasma}(T)} - V_0\right]}{\dfrac{\displaystyle\int_0^T C_{plasma}(t)\,dt}{C_{plasma}(T)}} \quad (4)$$

Considering V_0 and the SPIF known, K_i can be estimated using the value of $C_{tissue}(T)$ obtained from a single static scan. In effect, the plasma clearance at any site in the skeleton is calculated from a Patlak graph with just two data points (**Fig. 12A**). The right upper point is obtained from

Box 3
Advantages of SPIF

- Reliable measurement of the 0- to 60-minute terminal exponential from venous blood sampling
- Reliable estimation of bolus peak improves 0- to 60-minute curve fit to the Hawkins model
- Improved precision for measurements of K_i
- Enables K_i to be evaluated from static and dynamic scans
- Enables K_i to be evaluated at multiple sites from one injection
- Static scan method enables hip studies avoiding high bladder activity

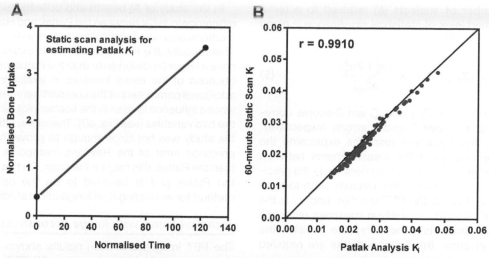

Fig. 12. Derivation of K_i using the static scan method.[41] The right upper point is based on a measurement of bone uptake from a single 5-minute static scan and the normalized uptake and normalized time are calculated in the same way as the Patlak plot (see **Fig. 7A**). The left lower point is the intercept of the graph and represents the population average volume of distribution of tracer at the measurement site. The value of K_i is obtained from the slope of the straight line through the two points. (*B*) Scatter plots for values of lumbar spine K_i obtained by the static scan method 60 minutes after tracer injection against the corresponding results from the Patlak plot method.

a single measurement of bone uptake from a static scan, whereas the left lower point is the intercept of the graph and represents the population average volume of distribution of tracer at that site. Based on Patlak plot data from dynamic scans, Siddique and colleagues[41] found mean values of $V_0 = 0.4$ for the spine and $V_0 = 0.2$ for the hip and other skeletal sites.

Fig. 12B shows the scatter plot for lumbar spine K_i values estimated using the static scan method at 60 minutes after injection against the results from the Patlak method. Because the value of k_4 is not zero, the ratio of the static scan K_i value to the Patlak plot K_i value obtained from the 10- to 60-minute dynamic scan data varies slightly with the timing of the static scan. Siddique and colleagues[41] found that the mean ratio reached a maximum of 1.008 (standard deviation, 0.013) approximately 30 minutes after injection and decreased to 0.967 (standard deviation, 0.015) by 60 minutes (**Fig. 13**). Like the Patlak method, the static scan method cannot be used to evaluate K_1.

Precision and Sensitivity

Measuring the precision errors of different approaches to [18]F NaF PET data analysis is important for comparing methods and determining the optimum technique.[40] Until the precision error is known, whether a measurement shows that real change has occurred is impossible to decide.[55] Furthermore, when planning research studies using

[18]F NaF PET, these must be properly powered to detect treatment-induced changes. If a study involves subjects that serve as their own controls with a baseline scan and a single follow-up scan,

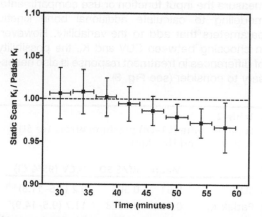

Fig. 13. Graph showing the mean ratio of the static scan measurement of lumbar spine K_i to the Patlak plot value for the [18]F NaF PET scan data shown in **Fig. 12B** plotted as a function of time after injection.[41] The error bars are ± 2 SDs. The static scan method provides accurate estimates of the Patlak plot K_i results between 30 and 60 minutes after injection. (*From* Siddique M, Blake GM, Frost ML, et al. Estimation of regional bone metabolism from whole-body ^{18}F-fluoride PET static images. Eur J Nucl Med Mol Imaging 2012;39:337–43; with permission from the European Association of Nuclear Medicine.)

the number of subjects (N) required to achieve a specified level of statistical significance is given by Equation 5[56]:

$$N = \left(Z_{\alpha/2} + Z_\beta\right)^2 \times \frac{(\sigma_b^2 + 2\sigma_p^2)}{\Delta_{treat}^2} \qquad (5)$$

In Equation 4, $Z_{\alpha/2}$ and Z_β are Z-scores corresponding to types 1 and 2 errors, respectively, Δ_{treat} is the treatment response expressing the average change in the measurements between baseline and the end of treatment, σ_p is the precision error expressing the random scan-to-scan precision error in the PET variable, and σ_b is the inherent biologic variability in treatment response between subjects. Therefore, the smaller the precision error, the fewer subjects are required for a study.

Table 2 lists mean values of lumbar spine SUV, Patlak K_i, and Hawkins K_i and their precision errors expressed as the root mean square standard deviation (RMS SD) and the percentage coefficient of variation (%CV) for each scan analysis method as reported by Al-beyatti and colleagues.[57] The %CVs were 9.2% for SUV, 11.7% for Patlak K_i and 14.5% for Hawkins K_i, although only the difference between SUV and the Hawkins method was statistically significant ($P = .003$). The finding that precision errors were smallest for SUV is expected given that this method only requires the measurement of bone uptake, and there is no need to measure the input function or use compartmental modeling to calculate additional bone kinetic parameters that add to the variability. However, in choosing between SUV and K_i, the possibility of differences in treatment response is also necessary to consider (see **Fig. 8**).

Table 2
Lumbar spine (L1–L4) precision errors for SUV, Patlak K_i, and Hawkins

	Mean	RMS SD	%CV (95% CI)
SUV	5.51	0.506	9.2 (7.5–11.8)[a,b]
Patlak K_i	0.024	0.0028	11.7 (9.5–14.9)[c]
Hawkins K_i	0.033	0.0048	14.5 (11.7–18.5)

Abbreviations: %CV, precision error expressed as percentage of the mean; K_i, plasma clearance to bone mineral (units: mL min^{-1} mL^{-1}); RMS SD, root mean square standard deviation; SUV, standardized uptake value.
[a] $P = .003$ versus Hawkins K_i.
[b] $P = .072$ versus Patlak K_i.
[c] $P = .096$ versus Hawkins K_i.
Data from Al-beyatti Y, Siddique M, Frost ML, et al. Precision of 18F-Fluoride PET skeletal kinetic studies in the assessment of bone metabolism. Osteoporos Int 2012. [Epub ahead of print]. DOI: 10.1007/s00198-011-1889-2.s.

In the study of Al-beyatti and colleagues,[57] the difference in %CV between the Patlak and Hawkins methods was not statistically significant ($P = .096$). Theoretically, the Hawkins method is expected to have a larger precision error than the Patlak method because of the errors involved in evaluating the additional parameters of the compartmental model, whose influence is seen in the scatter plot between the two variables (see **Fig. 6**B). Therefore, although the study was not large enough to prove that the precision error of the Hawkins method is larger than the Patlak, this may be the case. On this basis, the Patlak plot is believed to be the optimum method for evaluating K_i in longitudinal studies.[40]

Technical Issues with Image Reconstruction

The PET images and scan results shown in this review were all obtained using a 2D PET image acquisition protocol, and were reconstructed using filtered back projection (FBP) with a scatter correction (see **Box 2**). These choices are generally considered a safe option in the context of PET studies acquired primarily for image quantification. However, difficulties can arise with dynamic hip studies because of the accumulation of ^{18}F NaF in the urinary bladder, which is typically as much as 15% to 25% of the injected dose at the end of the 60-minute dynamic scan.[58] With this amount of radioactivity in the field of view, any slight movement by the subject can result in streak artifacts across transaxial scan planes through the bladder in images reconstructed using FBP. In some subjects, this effect is large enough to generate serious errors in quantitative measurements in hip ROIs intersected by these planes, particularly affecting the femoral neck. **Fig. 14** shows a similar case that occurred in the spine, in which intense retention of ^{18}F NaF in the renal calyces caused streaking artifacts in the transaxial planes intersecting L2 that distorted the bone TAC for this vertebra (see **Fig. 5**, Case 4). In the hip, these effects can be mitigated using the static scan K_i method described earlier, with the subject emptying their bladder immediately before scan acquisition, resulting in much-reduced activity in the field of view and a significant improvement in image quality. Image reconstruction using the ordered subset expectation maximization (OSEM) algorithm[59] may offer another method of reducing the streaking artifacts associated with FBP that is currently being investigated for the quantitative analysis of ^{18}F NaF PET studies.

^{18}F NAF PET STUDIES IN OSTEOPOROSIS
Treatment with Bisphosphonates

Bisphosphonates are antiresorptive agents,[9] and therefore the initiation of treatment leads to a rapid

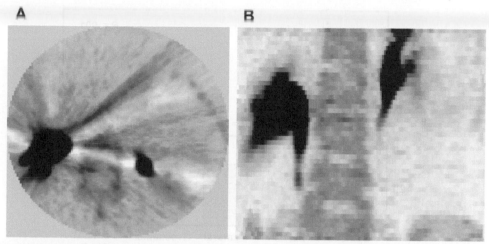

Fig. 14. (*A*) transaxial image through second lumbar vertebra, and (*B*) coronal ^{18}F NaF PET image of the lumbar spine in a subject with intense retention of tracer in the renal calyces. The streaking artifacts in (*A*) arise from reconstruction of the PET scan images using filtered back projection. The bone TAC for L2 is shown in Case 4 in **Fig. 5.**

decrease in biochemical markers of bone resorption, followed 1 or 2 months later by a reduction in bone formation markers.[16] Thus, after 2 or 3 months of treatment, ^{18}F NaF PET measurements would be expected to show a decrease in K_i and SUV values. The first study to examine this effect was reported by Frost and colleagues,[32] who performed dynamic PET scans of the lumbar spine in 18 postmenopausal women starting treatment with risedronate (see **Table 1**). On average, plasma clearance decreased by 18% from a mean figure of 0.033 mL min^{-1} mL^{-1} at baseline to 0.027 mL min^{-1} mL^{-1} after 6 months on risedronate ($P = .04$), whereas biochemical markers of bone formation and bone resorption decreased by 23% and 18%, respectively.

Equation 1 shows that values of K_i change either in response to a change in bone blood flow (K_1), or a change in the fraction of tracer transferred from the unbound bone pool to bone mineral $k_3/(k_2 + k_3)$, or both. The results of the risedronate study showed no significant change in K_1, but an 18% decrease in $k_3/(k_2 + k_3)$, suggesting that the primary effect of risedronate treatment was a decrease in the density of sites for tracer deposition in the bone mineral compartment, consistent with decreased osteoblastic activity. Frost and colleagues[32] did not report the changes in SUV, and therefore the treatment effects on bone uptake and bone plasma clearance cannot be compared in this study.

In another study using quantitative ^{18}F NaF PET to examine the effects of BP treatment on bone, Uchida and colleagues[43] reported a 14% decrease in SUV at the lumbar spine and a 24% decrease at the femoral neck in 24 postmenopausal women treated with alendronate for 12 months for glucocorticoid-induced osteoporosis. These authors did not measure plasma clearance, and therefore this study also does not give any information on the difference in treatment effect between K_i and SUV.

Treatment with Parathyroid Hormone

Teriparatide (recombinant human parathyroid hormone fragment rhPTH(1-34)) is one of the more potent treatments available for the prevention of osteoporotic fractures (see **Table 1**).[5] It acts through an anabolic mechanism to promote bone formation, resulting in a net positive bone balance.[10] Accretion of new bone on trabecular and cortical bone surfaces leads to improved bone microarchitecture with an associated increase in bone mineral density and reduction in fracture risk.[12–14,60,61] Hence, treatment with teriparatide would be expected to lead to increased values of SUV and K_i in all areas of the skeleton. A recent ^{18}F NaF PET study gave interesting new information that teriparatide has different effects at trabecular and cortical sites in the skeleton.[33] So large is the global effect of teriparatide on bone uptake across the whole skeleton that the treatment was found to change the arterial input function as the blood concentration of tracer declined more rapidly with time during the 60-minute scan because of the greater quantities of tracer being taken up by bone tissue (see **Fig. 7**B).[45]

In the study mentioned earlier, Frost and colleagues[33] used ^{18}F NaF PET to examine the

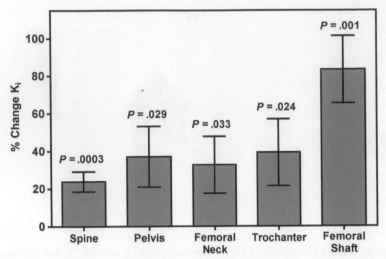

Fig. 15. Mean percentage change in regional bone ^{18}F NaF plasma clearance after 6 months of treatment with teriparatide at the lumbar spine, pelvis, femoral neck, trochanter, and femoral shaft.[33] Error bars are 1 standard error of the mean (SEM).

effect of 6 months of treatment on bone plasma clearance and SUV. At the end of a 60-minute dynamic scan of the lumbar spine, the subjects emptied their bladder and static scans were acquired to measure static scan K_i and SUV in the pelvis, hip, and femoral shaft. Baseline and follow-up scans were available for a total of 18 women. In the lumbar vertebral bodies plasma clearance increased on average by 24% from a mean figure of 0.035 mL min^{-1} mL^{-1} at baseline to 0.043 mL min^{-1} mL^{-1} ($P = .0003$) after 6 months of treatment. Other parameters in the Hawkins model were unchanged except for the fractional forward transfer of tracer to the bone mineral compartment [$k_3/(k_2 + k_3)$], which increased from 0.33 to 0.40 ($P = .0006$).

The static scan K_i measurements in the femoral shaft and hip showed evidence that teriparatide has different effects at different sites in the skeleton. In contrast to the 24% increase in K_i for trabecular bone in the lumbar vertebral bodies, values for cortical bone in the femoral shaft increased by 81% ($P = .001$) **(Fig. 15)** and were statistically significantly larger than the changes measured at the spine ($P = .005$). Changes in static scan K_i values in the femoral neck (+32.5%; $P = .033$), intertrochanteric region (+39.0%; $P = .024$), and pelvis (+36.8%; $P = .029$), all sites with a mixture of cortical and trabecular bone, were intermediate between those seen at the femoral shaft and spine (see **Fig. 15**).

In contrast to the 24% increase in lumbar spine K_i, at the end of the 60-minute dynamic scan, SUV at the lumbar spine increased by only 3.0%, a change that was not significantly different from

zero ($P = .84$). When the K_i and SUV changes were compared, a statistically significant difference in treatment effect was found at the spine ($P = .0013$). SUV changes in the proximal femur and pelvis were also smaller than those in K_i (femoral shaft: 37% vs 81%; intertrochanteric region: 20% vs 39%; pelvis: 11% vs 37%). As shown in **Fig. 8**, the difference in findings between the SUV and K_i results are explained by a 20% decrease in ^{18}F NaF plasma concentrations (see **Fig. 7**). It is clear, therefore, that teriparatide has different effects on different areas of the skeleton, with changes in trabecular bone at the spine being considerably smaller than for cortical bone at the femoral shaft. The unexpectedly large decrease in plasma concentrations is only explicable if the changes in the femoral shaft are typical of cortical bone across the whole skeleton.

SUMMARY

Quantitative ^{18}F NaF PET imaging provides a novel way to study bone metabolism that complements conventional measurements using bone turnover markers as a research tool to investigate new treatments for osteoporosis. Unlike bone markers that measure the integrated response to treatment across the whole skeleton, ^{18}F NaF PET can distinguish the changes occurring at sites of particular clinical interest, such as the hip and spine. Dynamic PET scans measure effective bone plasma flow and ^{18}F NaF bone plasma clearance, but, with a single injection, measurement sites are limited to the field of view of the PET scanner. In contrast, static PET scan images can be used to estimate plasma clearance at multiple sites throughout the skeleton with a single injection, provided venous blood samples are also taken. SUVs may also be measured but are partly responsive to the bone metabolic activity at sites other than the measurement site. As expected, treatment with a BP caused a decrease in bone plasma clearance, whereas treatment with teriparatide caused an increase. Teriparatide studies are of particular interest because they provide evidence that treatment with intermittent parathyroid hormone has different effects at different sites in the skeleton. Future studies may examine osteonecrosis of the jaw and atypical fractures of the femur to investigate underlying changes in bone metabolism.

REFERENCES

1. Storm T, Thamsborg G, Steiniche T, et al. Effect of intermittent cyclical etidronate therapy on bone mass and fracture rate in women with postmenopausal osteoporosis. N Engl J Med 1990;322:1265–71.
2. Black DM, Cummings SR, Karpf DB, et al. Randomised trial of the effect of alendronate on risk of fracture in women with existing vertebral fractures. Lancet 1996;348:1535–41.
3. Ettinger B, Black DM, Mitlak BH, et al. Reduction of vertebral fracture risk in postmenopausal women with osteoporosis treated with raloxifene: results from a 3-year randomised clinical trial. JAMA 1999; 282:637–45.
4. Harris ST, Watts NB, Genant HK, et al. Effects of risedronate treatment on vertebral and non-vertebral fractures in women with postmenopausal osteoporosis. JAMA 1999;282:1344–52.
5. Neer RM, Arnaud CD, Zanchetta JR, et al. Effect of recombinant human parathyroid hormone (1-34) fragment on spine and non-spine fractures and bone mineral density in postmenopausal osteoporosis. N Engl J Med 2001;344:1434–41.
6. Chesnut CH, Skag A, Christiansen C, et al. Effects of oral ibandronate administered daily or intermittently on fracture risk in postmenopausal osteoporosis. J Bone Miner Res 2004;19:1241–9.
7. Black DM, Delmas PD, Eastell R, et al. Once-yearly zoledronic acid for treatment of postmenopausal osteoporosis. N Engl J Med 2007;356:1809–22.
8. Cummings SR, San Martin J, McClung MR, et al. Denosumab for prevention of fractures in postmenopausal women with osteoporosis. N Engl J Med 2009;361:756–65.
9. Russell RG. Bisphosphonates: the first 40 years. Bone 2011;49:2–19.
10. McClung MR, San Martin J, Miller PD, et al. Opposite bone remodeling effects of teriparatide and alendronate in increasing bone mass. Arch Intern Med 2005;165:1762–8.
11. Dempster DW, Cosman F, Kurland ES, et al. Effects of daily treatment with parathyroid hormone on bone microarchitecture and turnover in patients with osteoporosis: a paired biopsy study. J Bone Miner Res 2001;16:1846–53.
12. Jiang Y, Zhao JJ, Mitlak BH, et al. Recombinant human parathyroid hormone (1-34) (teriparatide) improves both cortical and cancellous bone structure. J Bone Miner Res 2003;18:1932–41.
13. Arlot M, Meunier PJ, Boivin G, et al. Differential effects of teriparatide and alendronate on bone remodeling in postmenopausal women assessed by histomorphometric parameters. J Bone Miner Res 2005;20:1244–53.
14. Lindsay R, Zhou H, Cosman F, et al. Effects of a one-month treatment with PTH(1-34) on bone formation on cancellous, endocortical, and periosteal surfaces of the human ilium. J Bone Miner Res 2007;22:495–502.
15. Gruber R, Pietschmann P, Peterlik M. Introduction to bone development, remodelling and repair. In: Grampp S, editor. Radiology of osteoporosis. 2nd edition. Berlin: Springer; 2008. p. 1–23.
16. Garnero P, Weichung JS, Gineyts E, et al. Comparison of new biochemical markers of bone turnover in late postmenopausal osteoporotic women in response to alendronate treatment. J Clin Endocrinol Metab 1994;79:1693–700.
17. Glover SJ, Eastell R, McCloskey EV, et al. Rapid and robust response of biochemical markers of bone formation to teriparatide therapy. Bone 2009;45: 1053–8.
18. Hawkins RA, Choi Y, Huang SC, et al. Evaluation of the skeletal kinetics of fluorine-18-fluoride ion with PET. J Nucl Med 1992;33:633–42.
19. Moore AE, Blake GM, Taylor KA, et al. Changes observed in radionuclide bone scans during and after teriparatide treatment for osteoporosis. Eur J Nucl Med Mol Imaging 2012;39:326–36.
20. Blake GM, Park-Holohan S, Cook GJR, et al. Quantitative studies of bone with the use of 18F-fluoride and 99mTc-methylene diphosphonate. Semin Nucl Med 2001;31:28–49.
21. Messa C, Goodman WG, Hoh CK, et al. Bone metabolic activity measured with positron emission tomography and 18F-fluoride ion in renal osteodystrophy: correlation with bone histomorphometry. J Clin Endo Metab 1993;77:949–55.
22. Piert M, Zittel TT, Becker GA, et al. Assessment of porcine bone metabolism by dynamic 18F-fluoride PET: correlation with bone histomorphometry. J Nucl Med 2001;42:1091–100.
23. Blau M, Nagler W, Bender MA. Fluorine-18: a new isotope for bone scanning. J Nucl Med 1962;3: 332–4.
24. Grant FD, Fahey FH, Packard AB, et al. Skeletal PET with 18F-Fluoride: applying new technology to an old tracer. J Nucl Med 2008;49:68–78.

25. Li Y, Schiepers C, Lake R, et al. Clinical utility of ^{18}F-fluoride PET/CT in benign and malignant bone diseases. Bone 2012;50:128–39.

26. Czernin J, Satyamurthy N, Schiepers C. Molecular mechanisms of bone ^{18}F-NaF deposition. J Nucl Med 2010;51:1826–9.

27. Guillemart A, Besnard JC, Le Pape A, et al. Skeletal uptake of pyrophosphate labeled with technetium-95m and technetium-96, as evaluated by autoradiography. J Nucl Med 1978;19:895–9.

28. Schümichen C, Rempfle H, Wagner M, et al. The short-term fixation of radiopharmaceuticals in bone. Eur J Nucl Med 1979;4:423–8.

29. Einhorn TA, Vigorita VJ, Aaron A. Localization of technetium-99m methylene diphosphonate in bone using microautoradiography. J Orthop Res 1986;4:180–7.

30. Budd RS, Hodgson GS, Hare WS. The relation of radionuclide uptake by bone to the rate of calcium mineralization. I: experimental studies using [45]Ca, ^{32}P and [99]Tcm-MDP. Br J Radiol 1989;62:314–7.

31. Boivin G, Farlay D, Khebbab MT, et al. In osteoporotic women treated with strontium ranelate, strontium is located in bone formed during treatment with a maintained degree of mineralization. Osteoporos Int 2010;21:667–77.

32. Frost ML, Cook GJR, Blake GM, et al. A prospective study of risedronate on regional bone metabolism and blood flow at the lumbar spine measured by ^{18}F-fluoride positron emission tomography. J Bone Miner Res 2003;18:2215–22.

33. Frost ML, Siddique M, Blake GM, et al. Differential effects of teriparatide on regional bone formation using ^{18}F-fluoride positron emission tomography. J Bone Miner Res 2011;26:1002–11.

34. Taves DR. Electrophoretic mobility of serum fluoride. Nature 1968;220:582–3.

35. Schiepers C, Nuyts J, Bormans G, et al. Fluoride kinetics of the axial skeleton measured in vivo with fluorine-18-fluoride PET. J Nucl Med 1997;38:1970–6.

36. Cook GJ, Lodge MA, Marsden PK, et al. Non-invasive assessment of skeletal kinetics using fluorine-18 fluoride positron emission tomography: evaluation of image and population-derived arterial input functions. Eur J Nucl Med 1999;26:1424–9.

37. Installe J, Nzeusseu A, Bol A, et al. ^{18}F-fluoride PET for monitoring therapeutic response in Paget's disease of bone. J Nucl Med 2005;46:1650–8.

38. Wootton R, Doré C. The single-passage extraction of ^{18}F in rabbit bone. Clin Phys Physiol Meas 1986;7:333–43.

39. Piert M, Zittel TT, Machulla HJ, et al. Blood flow measurements with [15]OH$_2$O and ^{18}F-fluoride ion PET in porcine vertebrae. J Bone Miner Res 1998;13:1328–36.

40. Siddique M, Frost ML, Blake GM, et al. The precision and sensitivity of ^{18}F-fluoride PET for measuring regional bone metabolism: a comparison of quantification methods. J Nucl Med 2011;52:1748–55.

41. Siddique M, Blake GM, Frost ML, et al. Estimation of regional bone metabolism from whole-body ^{18}F-fluoride PET static images. Eur J Nucl Med Mol Imaging 2012;39:337–43.

42. Akaike H. A new look at the statistical model identification. IEEE Trans Automat Contr 1974;19:716–23.

43. Uchida K, Nakajima H, Miyazaki T, et al. Effects of alendronate on bone metabolism in glucocorticoid-induced osteoporosis measured by ^{18}F-fluoride PET: a prospective study. J Nucl Med 2009;50:1808–14.

44. Keyes JW. SUV: standard uptake or silly useless value? J Nucl Med 1995;36:1836–9.

45. Blake GM, Siddique M, Frost ML, et al. Radionuclide studies of bone metabolism: do bone uptake and bone plasma clearance provide equivalent measurements of bone turnover? Bone 2011;49:537–42.

46. Gnanasegaran G, Moore AE, Blake GM, et al. Atypical Paget's disease with quantitative assessment of tracer kinetics. Clin Nucl Med 2007;32:765–9.

47. Blake GM, Zivanovic MA, McEwan AJ, et al. [89]Sr therapy: strontium kinetics in disseminated carcinoma of the prostate. Eur J Nucl Med 1986;12:447–54.

48. Blake GM, Frost ML, Fogelman I. Quantitative radionuclide studies of bone. J Nucl Med 2009;50:1747–50.

49. Piert M, Machulla HJ, Jahn M, et al. Coupling of porcine bone blood flow and metabolism in high-turnover bone disease measured by ^{15}O]H$_2$O and ^{18}F]fluoride ion positron emission tomography. Eur J Nucl Med Mol Imaging 2002;29:907–14.

50. Renkin EM. Transport of potassium-42 from blood to tissue in isolated mammalian skeletal muscles. Am J Physiol 1959;197:1205–10.

51. Crone C. The permeability of capillaries in various organs as determined by the use of the 'indicator diffusion' method. Acta Physiol Scand 1963;58:292–305.

52. Chen K, Bandy D, Reiman E, et al. Noninvasive quantification of the cerebral metabolic rate for glucose using positron emission tomography, 18F-fluoro-2-deoxyglucose, the Patlak method, and an image-derived input function. J Cereb Blood Flow Metab 1998;18:716–23.

53. Puri T, Blake GM, Siddique M, et al. Validation of new image-derived arterial input functions at the aorta using 18F-fluoride positron emission tomography. Nucl Med Commun 2011;32:486–95.

54. Puri T, Blake GM, Frost ML, et al. Validation of image-derived arterial input functions at the femoral artery using 18F-fluoride positron emission tomography. Nucl Med Commun 2011;32:808–17.

55. Bonnick SL, Johnston C, Kleerekoper M, et al. Importance of precision in bone density measurements. J Clin Densitom 2001;4:105–10.

56. Sowers MF, Karvonen-Gutierrez CA. Epidemiological methods in studies of osteoporosis. In: Marcus R, Feldman D, Nelson DA, et al, editors. Osteoporosis. 3rd edition. Burlington (MA): Elsevier Academic Press; 2007. p. 645–65.

57. Al-beyatti Y, Siddique M, Frost ML, et al. Precision of 18F-Fluoride PET skeletal kinetic studies in the assessment of bone metabolism. Osteoporos Int 2012. [Epub ahead of print].

58. Park-Holohan SJ, Blake GM, Fogelman I. Quantitative studies of bone using ^{18}F-fluoride and ^{99}mTc-methylene diphosphonate: evaluation of renal and whole blood kinetics. Nucl Med Commun 2001;22: 1037–44.

59. Boellaard R, van Lingen A, Lammertsma AA. Experimental and clinical evaluation of iterative reconstruction (OSEM) in dynamic PET: quantitative characteristics and effects on kinetic modeling. J Nucl Med 2001;42:808–17.

60. Chen P, Miller PD, Recker R, et al. Increases in BMD correlate with improvements in bone microarchitecture with teriparatide treatment in postmenopausal women with osteoporosis. J Bone Miner Res 2007; 22:1173–80.

61. Dobnig H, Sipos A, Jiang Y, et al. Early changes in biochemical markers of bone formation correlate with improvements in bone structure during teriparatide therapy. J Clin Endocrinol Metab 2005;90:3970–7.

Pediatric Bone Scanning
Clinical Indication of 18F NaF PET/CT

Laura A. Drubach, MD

KEYWORDS

- Fluorine-18 NaF • Positron emission tomography • Bone scintigraphy • Stress fractures

KEY POINTS

- Fluorine-18 (18F)-labeled sodium fluoride provides an excellent alternative to 99mTc MDP for radio-nuclide bone scintigraphy in the evaluation of pediatric bone pathology.
- The excellent image quality obtained with 18F NaF PET makes this radiopharmaceutical the best option for evaluation of bone trauma in children.
- 18F NaF PET shows excellent sensitivity for detection of rib fractures, but lower sensitivity in identifying classic methaphyseal lesion fractures in cases of child abuse.

INTRODUCTION

From the time of its introduction in 1962, fluorine-18 (18F) NaF has been recognized as a nearly ideal radiopharmaceutical agent for skeletal imaging.[1] Imaging with 18F NaF positron emission tomography (PET) offers several technological advantages compared with conventional scintigraphy using 99mTc- methylene diphosphate (MDP), including more rapid bone uptake and faster blood clearance, combined with the higher spatial resolution, greater sensitivity, and improved image quality that PET imaging provides.[2] These characteristics are of particular importance when imaging children; the structures being imaged are smaller than in adults, and optimal evaluation of many pediatric bone imaging applications requires a technique that provides excellent resolution.

Imaging of children who are being evaluated for nonaccidental trauma requires high image quality to be able to detect corner fractures, a characteristic type of fractures seen in child abuse. Patients being evaluated for back pain, suspected end plate spine injuries, or subtle bone metastasis from neuroblastoma, are just some examples in which a technique with the greatest possible resolution is important.

Bone scan continues to be a frequent procedure in pediatric nuclear medicine.[3] The most common indications for bone scans in children are the evaluation of trauma, either accidental or nonaccidental, evaluation of sports-related bony injuries, survey for bone metastatic disease in patients with a known malignancy, and the evaluation of osteomyelitis.[3] The bone scan is particularly important in the evaluation of young children, because localization of the abnormality by clinical symptomatology alone is often difficult. The ability to image the entire skeleton without additional radiation burden to the patient is of great importance in this age group. 18F NaF PET can be used effectively in children in all typical indications for which the standard bone scan is used.

PHARMACOKINETICS

18F NaF has a biodistribution similar to that of 99mTc-MDP, but its lower protein binding in blood results in more rapid single passage extraction by bone, allowing for earlier image acquisition.[4,5] Imaging can be started as early as 30 to 45 minutes after administration of tracer, as opposed to the 2 to 3 hours required by MDP. In addition to faster uptake, there is greater extraction of 18F NaF by

Department of Radiology, Children's Hospital Boston, 300 Longwood Avenue, Boston, MA 02115, USA
E-mail address: Laura.Drubach@childrens.harvard.edu

PET Clin 7 (2012) 293–301
doi:10.1016/j.cpet.2012.04.004

bone than is seen with diphosphonate compounds, so that the concentration of ^{18}F NaF in bone is approximately 2 times greater than ^{99}Tc MDP.[2] The combination of lower remaining soft tissue tracer activity and higher bone extraction of ^{18}F NaF produces images with a higher target-to-background ratio and better image contrast than with MDP imaging. ^{18}F NaF clears rapidly from the blood and is excreted from the body via the kidneys.[3]

The physical characteristics of PET imaging also provide substantial advantages for ^{18}F NaF imaging in comparison to ^{99m}Tc labeled single-photon techniques. The intrinsic spatial resolution of current PET imaging is approximately 4 to 5 mm compared with the 10 to 15 mm obtainable with either planar or tomographic gamma camera imaging using ^{99m}Tc.

The normal biodistribution of ^{18}F NaF in children varies with age, in the same manner as is seen with MDP, with greater uptake in the growth centers (**Fig. 1**).

DOSIMETRY

The effective dose for ^{18}F NaF is 0.089 mrem/mCi (0.024 mSv/MBq) compared with an effective dose for ^{99m}Tc-MDP of 0.021 mrem/mCi (0.0057 mSv/MBq).[2]

The radiation dose per mCi from ^{18}F NaF is thus greater than from ^{99m}Tc-MDP, with a 68% greater absorbed dose per millicurie when ^{18}F NaF is used in comparison with ^{99m}Tc-MDP.[2] Despite this less favorable dosimetry, good quality ^{18}F NaF imaging can be effectively performed using a smaller administered dosage than is typically employed for MDP, resulting in an actual radiation absorbed dose that is equivalent to that received from standard single-photon imaging (**Table 1**).[6]

When imaging with ^{18}F NaF, the target organ is the urinary bladder, as opposed to ^{99m}Tc-MDP, where the target is the bone marrow.[6] With good hydration and frequent urination, the radiation exposure of the patient can be decreased considerably.

The addition of a computed tomography (CT) scan to the PET/CT, either as an attenuation correction or diagnostic imaging, also increases the radiation exposure to the patient. In most cases, bone imaging without CT is sufficient information for diagnosis, employing CT only in selected situations.[7]

TECHNIQUE

PET imaging with ^{18}NaF can be performed either as a whole-body scan or with limited imaging of the region of interest, according to the indication of the study. Acquisition of images can be performed either using a 2-dimensional or 3-dimensional mode.

Imaging can begin as early as 30 to 45 minutes following tracer injection, although a longer delay

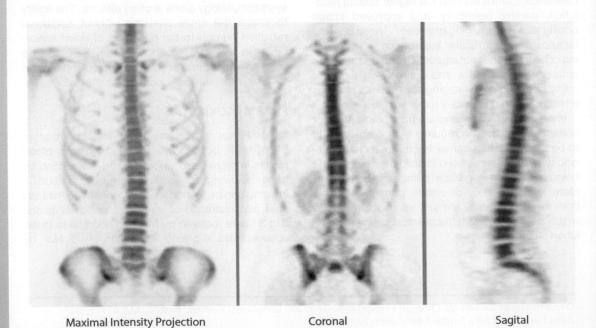

Maximal Intensity Projection   Coronal   Sagital

Fig. 1. Normal ^{18}F NaF PET in a 15-year-old with low back pain.

Table 1
Radiation dosimetry of ^{99m}Tc-MDP scintigraphy versus ^{18}F-labeled NaF PET

	Adult (70 kg)	15 y (55 kg)	10 y (32 kg)	5 y (19 kg)	1 y (9.8 kg)
99mTc-MDP[a]					
Administered activity (MBq)	518	407	237	141	73
Effective dose in mSv/MBq (mSv)	0.0057 (3.0)	0.0070 (2.8)	0.0110 (2.6)	0.0140 (2.0)	0.0270 (2.0)
Bladder wall in mGy/MBq (mGy)	0.048 (24.9)	0.060 (24.4)	0.088 (20.9)	0.073 (10.3)	0.130 (9.5)
Bone surfaces (mGy)	0.063 (32.6)	0.082 (33.4)	0.130 (30.8)	0.220 (31.0)	0.53 (38.7)
Red marrow (mGy)	0.0092 (4.8)	0.010 (4.1)	0.017 (4.0)	0.033 (4.7)	0.067 (4.9)
18F-labeled NaF y					
Administered activity (MBq)	148	116	68	40	21
Effective dose in mSv/MBq (mSv)	0.027 (4.0)	0.034 (3.9)	0.052 (3.5)	0.086 (3.4)	0.170 (3.6)
Bladder wall in mGy/MBq (mGy)	0.22 (32.6)	0.27 (31.3)	0.40 (27.2)	0.61 (24.4)	1.10 (23.1)
Bone surfaces in mGy/MBq (mGy)	0.040 (5.9)	0.050 (5.8)	0.079 (5.4)	0.130 (5.2)	0.300 (6.3)
Red marrow in mGy/MBq (mGy)	0.040 (5.9)	0.053 (6.1)	0.088 (6.0)	0.180 (7.2)	0.380 (8.0)

Abbreviation: MBq, megabequerel.
Derived from International Commission on Radiological Protection (ICRP) Report 53. Ann ICRP 1987;17:74.
Values in parentheses are doses in mGy (mSv for effective dose) for administered activity listed in table for that patient size.
[a] Derived from ICRP Report 80. Ann ICRP 1999;28:75.

of 60 to 90 minutes will also produce images of high quality. The recommended dosage of ^{18}NaF in the pediatric population is 60 μCi/kg (2.2 MBq/kg), with a minimum of 300 μCi (11.1 MBq) and a maximum of 4 mCi (148 MBq).[2,8] Good hydration is recommended, with frequent voiding to minimize radiation dose, particularly to the bladder.

Unlike with fluorodeoxyglucose imaging, the high bone-to-soft tissue ratio of ^{18}F NaF bone scanning allows good quality PET images to be acquired without the use of attenuation correction.[2] Eliminating the CT attenuation correction acquisition minimizes radiation exposure to the patient, an especially important issue in pediatric imaging. Nonattenuation corrected images occasionally suffer from streak artifact resulting from intense renal uptake. This artifact can be minimized by ensuring good hydration and by allowing a longer interval from injection to imaging of 60 minutes and frequent bladder emptying. In selected cases, the acquisition of diagnostic-quality CT images may be useful, although registration and fusion of ^{18}F NaF images with existing, previously acquired CT or magnetic resonance imaging (MRI) can be performed.

When imaging toddlers or young children, sedation may be needed in some cases. Very young infants will commonly fall asleep and remain F immobile if fed just before imaging. Other than in extraordinary circumstances, sedation of older children and adolescents is not needed.

INDICATIONS

In the past decade, the clinical utility of ^{18}F NaF PET bone scans has been demonstrated by numerous studies that were mainly performed in the adult population. Most of these studies were done in patients with various oncologic diagnoses being evaluated for metastatic disease.[9,10] ^{18}F NaF PET was found to be sensitive in the detection of metastasis from a number of tumors such as prostate, breast, lung, and thyroid cancer. In children ^{18}F NaF PET has been studied in benign skeletal disorders and has proven to be of value in the evaluation of back pain, detection of bone trauma in sports-related injuries,[6,11–13] or injuries due to child abuse.[14] In young adults, ^{18}F NaF PET has also been found useful in the evaluation of condylar hyperplasia.[15]

The Society of Nuclear Medicine has recently published practice guidelines for the performance and interpretation of [18]F NaF PET.[2] These guidelines conclude that [18]F NaF may be appropriate for a number of benign and malignant indications.

Sports-Related Bone Injuries

Back pain or other suspected stress injuries are important indications for skeletal scintigraphy using [18]F NaF PET in children and young adults.[11]

The value of imaging with [18]F NaF in bone trauma in general has been proven in an experimental animal model, where it was found that stress fractures produced an increase in the uptake of [18]F NaF and that the uptake was proportional to the level of the initial bony damage.[7] The increased uptake was seen as early as 1 day after a loading injury, with peak uptake at approximately 1 week after injury, providing a rational basis for the use of [18]F NaF PET in trauma and sports injuries.

A review of the [18]F NaF PET studies performed in 94 children and young adults referred with symptoms of back pain showed that this technique could be effectively used in this population. This study revealed a possible cause for back pain in 55% of patients. The diagnoses detected by [18]F NaF PET included pars interarticularis/pedicle stress (34%), spinous process injury (16%), vertebral body ring apophyseal injury (14%), stress at

a transitional vertebra–sacral articulation (7%), and sacroiliac joint inflammation/stress (3%).[12]

In another study, 15 patients also referred with low back pain underwent [18]F NaF PET and concurrent CT imaging. In this group of patients, an abnormality was found in 10 patients: 4 cases of spondylolysis, 3 frank fractures (2 of the transverse process and 1 of the facet), 2 osteoid osteomas, 1 osteitis pubis, 1 sacroiliitis, and 2 herniated disks. Three patients presented with 2 coexisting pathologies.[13] [18]F NaF PET-CT was thus able to detect spinal lesions with high diagnostic accuracy in adolescents with back pain.

Due to its high image resolution, [18]F NaF PET is very sensitive for detection of end plate injuries, an abnormality difficult to diagnose on a conventional bone scan even if single-photon emission CT (SPECT) is performed (**Fig. 2**). Other abnormalities that have been detected with [18]F NaF PET are transverse process fractures, spine and spinous process fractures, spine compression fractures, and pelvis stress fractures (**Fig. 3**).[11] The high image quality of [18]F NaF PET often allows for confident diagnosis in these cases.

In another study performed in 2008, 67 patients with back pain and negative radiograph, CT, or MRI were referred to [18]F NaF PET/CT. Among the main group, a subset of 25 patients had previous spine surgery consisting of laminectomy or diskectomy (17 patients) and lumbar fusion (8 patients). The [18]F NaF PET/CT showed abnormal uptake in the spine in 56 patients, with an

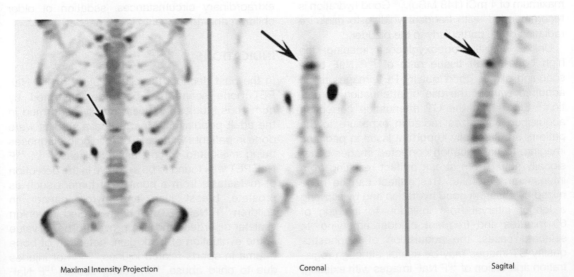

Maximal Intensity Projection   Coronal   Sagital

Fig. 2. 15-year-old female dancer with midback pain: [18]F NaF PET shows increased uptake in the superior anterior border of the T-12 vertebral body (*arrows*), suggestive of end-plate stress injury.

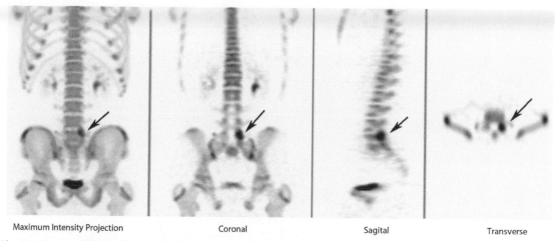

| Maximum Intensity Projection | Coronal | Sagital | Transverse |

Fig. 3. 15-year-old boy with low back pain on extension. Pars interarticularis stress fracture is seen on ^{18}F NaF PET (*arrows*).

overall detection ability of 84%. Facet joints were at the site of abnormality in 25 cases. One-third (36%) of the patients showed multiple positive uptake in both facet joints and disc areas (20 of 56 patients). In 42 patients who did not have a surgical procedure in the spine, ^{18}F NaF PET/ CT showed a source of pain in 88% of the studies. In the 25 patients with prior lumbar fusion or laminectomy, ^{18}F NaF PET/CT showed abnormal uptake in 76% of patients.[16]

It has been established that tomographic imaging improves the rate of detection of spine trauma in sport-related injuries,[17] and the superior resolution and localizing capabilities of ^{18}F NaF PET imaging provides theoretical advantages in the detection of inflicted spinal lesions in comparison to either conventional planar or SPECT bone scintigraphy.

Bone Trauma—Child Abuse

^{18}F NaF PET is of particular value in the evaluation of trauma related to child abuse.[14] Several types of fractures and patterns of fractures should arouse high suspicion for child abuse, such as the detection of multiple fractures at different stages of healing, multiple rib fractures, detection of classic methaphyseal lesion (CML), which is a series of microfractures across the metaphysis of the long bones, and posterior rib fractures.

The sensitivity of standard ^{99m}Tc labeled MDP bone scanning for the detection of fractures varies greatly depending on the location and type of fractures.[18] The sensitivity of Tc99m MDP for detection of fractures in child abuse was evaluated in a study performed in 2003 in which the

effectiveness of detection of fractures of the skeletal survey and conventional bone scintigraphy with Tc99m MDP was compared in 30 children being evaluated for child abuse.[19]

The total number of fractures identified on conventional bone scan was 64, while skeletal survey identified 77 fractures. Rib fractures represented 48% of the fractures identified by both techniques. CML, which is a typical fracture seen in cases of child abuse, was present in 20 cases. Conventional bone scan was able to detect only 35% of these fractures.[19]

Given the limitations of traditional MDP bone imaging in suspected child abuse, a technique with better resolution and sensitivity such as ^{18}F NaF PET is desirable to be able to detect these fractures.

In a recent study using ^{18}F NaF PET, the sensitivity for detection of CML was 67%, a substantial improvement over the previously described using standard ^{99m}Tc-MDP bone scan imaging.[14] This study evaluated the sensitivities of the baseline skeletal surveys and ^{18}F NaF PET when compared with a gold standard of the baseline skeletal survey plus the follow-up skeletal survey performed 2 weeks later, for detection of fractures in 22 children younger than 2 years. It was found that PET had a higher sensitivity for detection of fractures than the baseline skeletal survey in all fractures with exception of CML (**Fig. 4, Table 2**). ^{18}F NaF PET was particularly valuable in the detection of rib fractures, which are the most common fractures found in child abuse, with an overall sensitivity of 92% versus 68% for initial skeletal survey. ^{18}F NaF PET was also able to detect posterior rib fractures, which are very difficult to detect on radiography (**Fig. 5**).

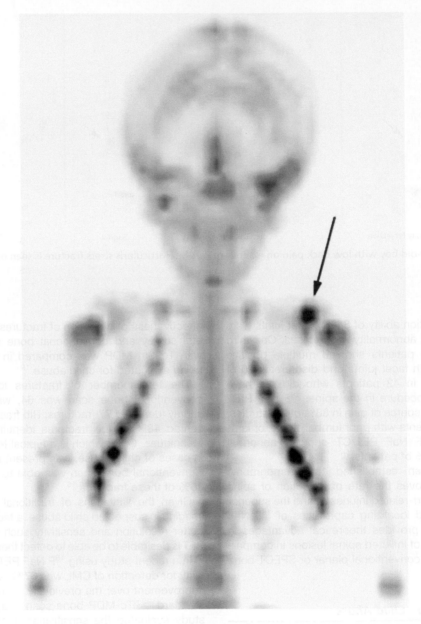

Coronal

Fig. 4. 9-month-old not moving left arm. ¹⁸F NaF PET shows fracture of the acromium (*arrow*).

Given the superior performance of ¹⁸NaF PET for the detection of rib fractures and other potential advantages over initial skeletal survey, the use of both techniques at baseline would likely increase the yield of imaging during the critical early assessment of children in selected cases of suspected abuse.

Condylar Hyperplasia

Unilateral condylar hyperplasia is a disorder that occurs most typically in adolescents and young adults. It is characterized by the overgrowth of 1 side of the temporomandibular joint, leading to significant asymmetry in the facial features in addition to significant dental problems related to mouth malocclusion. The optimal treatment is the surgical resection of the overgrowing condyle after all growth has ended.

Standard bone scintigraphy has been used extensively in an attempt to identify the time of cessation of condylar growth that would indicate the appropriate time for surgical repair. ¹⁸F NaF

Table 2
Sensitivity/specificity using the baseline plus follow-up skeletal survey as a gold standard in evaluation of child abuse

	PET	Baseline Skeletal Survey
All fractures	85%/97%	72%/98%
Thorax	92%/96%	68%/98%
Post-ribs	93%/93%	73%/99%
CML	67%/99%	80%/100%

PET was found to be able to correctly identify condylar hyperplasia in 5 patients studied, and the results of the scintigraphy correlated with the operative findings in all patients.[15]

Benign and Malignant Bone Lesions

Osteoid osteoma is a benign bone tumor that presents with a characteristic bone pain that is worse at night. Pain is generated by the secretion of prostaglandins by the tumor, producing localized pain. The diagnosis of osteoid osteoma may be suspected based upon symptoms, or the lesion may be found during a broader evaluation for possible sports-related injuries.[11,13] The scan appearance of an osteoid osteoma using [18]F NaF PET is similar to the appearance on a conventional bone scan, with increased uptake in the central nidus. [18]F NaF PET often gives a higher resolution of the location of the nidus, particularly when lesions are localized in the spine. Correlation with concurrently obtained CT may help with improved specificity of the findings on [18]F NaF PET.

In contrast with the vast publications looking at bone metastasis from different tumors in the adult population, there are to date no reports of the use of [18]F NaF PET in the pediatric population. It seems reasonable to speculate that [18]F NaF PET would also be useful for metastatic evaluation in pediatric oncologic disorders, but this currently remains in the realm of conjecture.

[18]F NaF PET was found to be sensitive in the detection of both osteoblastic and osteolytic primary bone lesions.[9,20] This may be a good characteristic to evaluate lytic processes commonly seen in children, such as eosinophilic granuloma (**Fig. 6**). Further studies evaluating the role of [18]F NaF PET in malignant disease in pediatrics are needed.

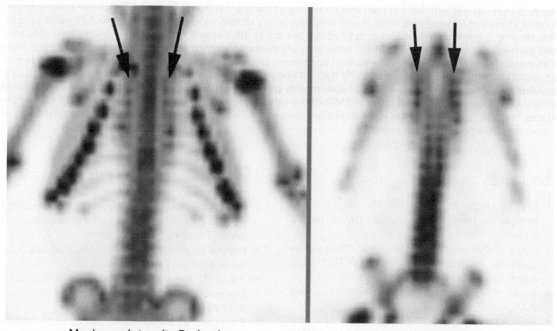

Maximum Intensity Projection   Coronal

Fig. 5. 3-month-old boy being evaluated for child abuse. Skeletal survey of the posterior ribs was negative. [18]F NaF PET performed 2 days after the skeletal survey showed multiple fractures at different thoracic levels (*arrows*) in the posterior ribs.

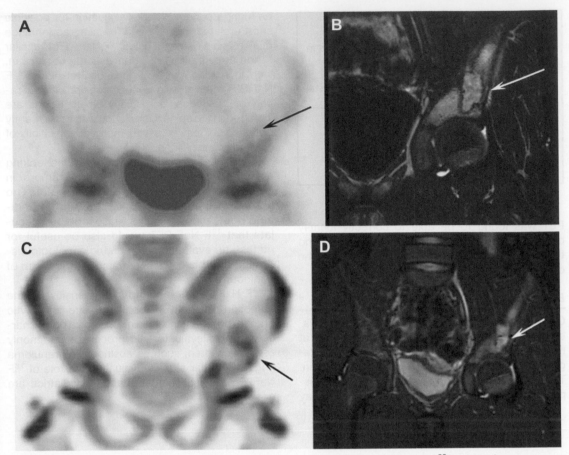

Fig. 6. 8-year-old girl with left hip pain and no history of trauma. (*A*) Planar image of ^{99m}Tc MDP bone scan performed at presentation of symptoms shows only very subtle diffuse increased uptake in the left pelvis (*arrow*). This finding is not characteristic of a defined disease entity. (*B*) Coronal fast spin echo (FSE) T2 fat-saturated MRI performed 1 month after the initial bone scan (*A*) shows a sharply marginated lesion within the left ilium with marked surrounding edema. The patient underwent a needle biopsy of this lesion that proved to be hystiocytosis. (*C*) maximum intensity projection ^{18}F NaF PET image of the pelvis shows increased uptake in the left supraacetabular iliac bone (*arrow*). The area of abnormality seen on ^{18}F NaF PET is better defined than on the initial bone scan. (*D*) Coronal FSE T2 fat saturated MRI of the pelvis performed 1 month after the ^{18}F NaF PET (*C*) demonstrates that the lytic lesion in the left acetabulum (*arrow*) has improved since the MRI done at presentation of symptoms (*B*), with less edema present.

REFERENCES

1. Blau M, Nagler W, Bender MA. Fluorine-18: a new isotope for bone scanning. J Nucl Med 1962;3: 332–4.

2. Segall G, Delbeke D, Stabin MG, et al. SNM practice guideline for sodium 18F-fluoride PET/CT bone scans 1.0. J Nucl Med 2010;51:1813–20.

3. Nadel HR. Bone scan update. Semin Nucl Med 2007;37:332–9.

4. Park-Holohan SJ, Blake GM, Fogelman I. Quantitative studies of bone using (18)F-fluoride and (99m) Tc-methylene diphosphonate: evaluation of renal and whole-blood kinetics. Nucl Med Commun 2001;22:1037–44.

5. Blau M, Ganatra R, Bender MA. 18 F-fluoride for bone imaging. Semin Nucl Med 1972;2:31–7.

6. Grant FD, Fahey FH, Packard AB, et al. Skeletal PET with 18F-fluoride: applying new technology to an old tracer. J Nucl Med 2008;49:68–78.

7. Brenner AI, Koshy J, Morey J, et al. The bone scan. Semin Nucl Med 2012;42:11–26.

8. Treves ST, Parisi MT, Gelfand MJ. Pediatric radiopharmaceutical doses: new guidelines. Radiology 2011;261:347–9.

9. Even-Sapir E, Metser U, Flusser G, et al. Assessment of malignant skeletal disease: initial experience with 18F-fluoride PET/CT and comparison between 18F-fluoride PET and 18F-fluoride PET/CT. J Nucl Med 2004;45:272–8.

10. Schirrmeister H, Buck A, Guhlmann A, et al. Anatomical distribution and sclerotic activity of bone metastases from thyroid cancer assessed with F-18 sodium fluoride positron emission tomography. Thyroid 2001;11:677–83.

11. Drubach LA, Connolly SA, Palmer EL 3rd. Skeletal scintigraphy with 18F-NaF PET for the evaluation of bone pain in children. AJR Am J Roentgenol 2011; 197:713–9.

12. Lim R, Fahey FH, Drubach LA, et al. Early experience with fluorine-18 sodium fluoride bone PET in young patients with back pain. J Pediatr Orthop 2007;27:277–82.

13. Ovadia D, Metser U, Lievshitz G, et al. Back pain in adolescents: assessment with integrated 18F-fluoride positron emission tomography–computed tomography. J Pediatr Orthop 2007;27:90–3.

14. Drubach LA, Johnston PR, Newton AW, et al. Skeletal trauma in child abuse: detection with 18F-NaF PET. Radiology 2010;255:173–81.

15. Laverick S, Bounds G, Wong WL. [18F]-fluoride positron emission tomography for imaging condylar hyperplasia. Br J Oral Maxillofac Surg 2009;47: 196–9.

16. Gamie S, El-Maghraby T. The role of PET/CT in evaluation of facet and disc abnormalities in patients with low back pain using (18)F-Fluoride. Nucl Med Rev Cent East Eur 2008;11:17–21.

17. Han LJ, Au-Yong TK, Tong WC, et al. Comparison of bone single-photon emission tomography and planar imaging in the detection of vertebral metastases in patients with back pain. Eur J Nucl Med 1998;25:635–8.

18. Kleinman PK. Skeletal trauma: general considerations. In: Kleinman PK, editor. Diagnostic imaging of child abuse. 2nd edition. St Louis (MO): Mosby; 1998. p. 8–25.

19. Mandelstam SA, Cook D, Fitzgerald M, et al. Complementary use of radiological skeletal survey and bone scintigraphy in detection of bony injuries in suspected child abuse. Arch Dis Child 2003;88: 387–90 [discussion: 90].

20. Bhargava P, Hanif M, Nash C. Whole-body F-18 sodium fluoride PET-CT in a patient with renal cell carcinoma. Clin Nucl Med 2008;33:894–5.

^{18}F NaF PET/CT in the Assessment of Metastatic Bone Disease
Comparison with Specific PET Tracers

Mohsen Beheshti, MD, FEBNM*, Werner Langsteger, MD

KEYWORDS

- Skeletal metastases • ^{18}F NaF PET • Fluorodeoxyglucose • Choline derivatives
- Specific PET tracers

KEY POINTS

- Specific PET tracers such as FDG, 11C-& ^{18}F Choline show promising results especially in the early detection of metastatic bone disease and therapy monitoring but inconsistent findings were seen in densely sclerotic bone lesions especially after therapy.
- ^{18}F NaF PET demonstrates higher sensitivity than ^{18}F-FDG and FCH PET for detection of bone metastases. However, ^{18}F-FDG and FCH PET have shown the potential to become "one stop diagnostic procedures" for detecting both bone and soft tissue disease.
- In patients with suspicious sclerotic lesions but negative ^{18}F-FCH and FDG PET, a second bone seeking agent (eg, ^{18}F NaF) is suggested.
- There is insufficient data about other PET tracers such as Acetate derivatives, 11C Methionine, ^{18}F-FDHT, and ^{18}F-FES available to draw conclusions concerning their potential value in the assessment of bone metastases.

BONE SCANNING

Bone is among the most common locations of metastasis, and therefore represents an important clinical target for diagnosis and follow-up in patients with cancer. Bone metastases have been reported in about 350,000 patients in the United States each year.[14–16] In the pathogenesis of bone metastases, proliferated tumor cells interact with the local microenvironment in the bone, stimulating or inhibiting osteoclast and osteoblast activity. Noninvasive imaging methods monitor molecular, functional, and morphologic changes in the skeletal system.

Nuclear imaging modalities, particularly with bone scintigraphy, have proved the mainstay of detection of bony disease for more than 40 years. Bone scanning with ^{99m}Tc-labeled diphosphonates

relies on the detection of pathologic osteoblastic response elicited from malignant cells. This technique offers the advantage of whole-body examination, low cost, availability, and high sensitivity; however, it suffers from relatively low specificity.

The addition of single-photon emission computed tomography (SPECT) to bone scintigraphy has markedly improved its diagnostic benefit. Although the accuracy of SPECT is significantly higher than that of planar scintigraphy, characterization of anatomic localization and morphologic changes with the upcoming combined SPECT/ computed tomography (CT) significantly improves the diagnostic accuracy of this modality.

PET, a modality with higher spatial resolution than that of SPECT, can be particularly helpful in detecting small lesions. Moreover, PET imaging

Department of Nuclear Medicine and Endocrinology, PET/CT Center LINZ, St Vincent's Hospital, Seilerstaette 4, A-4020, Linz, Austria
* Corresponding author.
E-mail address: mohsen.beheshti@bhs.at

PET Clin 7 (2012) 303–314
doi:10.1016/j.cpet.2012.04.002
1556-8598/12/$ – see front matter © 2012 Elsevier Inc. All rights reserved.

using various specific radiotracers has the advantage of detecting malignant lesions in both bone and soft tissues. PET imaging has also shown promise for early detection of bone marrow infiltration as well as for diagnosing lytic bony metastases.

In transiting to the clinical situation, these novel methods can be also reliably used to monitor therapy response.

Skeletal imaging using ^{18}F-labeled sodium fluoride ([18]F NaF) was first described in 1962.[17] With the introduction of gamma cameras it was replaced by ^{99m}Tc-labeled diphosphonates such as methylene diphosphonate (MDP), now the most commonly used bone-seeking substance.

With improvements in new PET scanners high-resolution imaging of bone became a reality, therefore [18]F NaF was reintroduced for clinical and research investigations.

Although only a few studies compare [18]F NaF with ^{99m}Tc-MDP for the diagnosis of bone metastases, [18]F NaF PET seems to be more sensitive than conventional bone scanning,[18] showing a higher contrast between normal and abnormal tissue and with the potential for the detection of additional lesions, especially in the spine.[18–25]

[18]F NaF diffuses through the capillaries into the extracellular fluid followed by a slow exchange of hydroxyl ions in the hydroxylapatite, hence indicating the rate of bone turnover.[25] [18]F NaF offers substantially higher sensitivity and resolution than that of Tc-labeled tracers because of its higher bony extraction as well as faster blood excretion.[25]

At present there are numerous novel molecular imaging agents potentially available for the assessment of bone metastases and different cancers.

This review assesses the role of PET in the imaging of skeletal metastases from various tumors, focusing on the specific PET tracers (fluorodeoxyglucose, choline derivatives, and so forth) in comparison with [18]F NaF as a nonspecific bone-seeking PET agent.

^{18}F-FLUORO-2-DEOXY-D-GLUCOSE

[18]F-Fluoro-2-deoxy-D-glucose (FDG) is the most common PET radiotracer in clinical use. FDG is transported into tumor cells by the glucose transporter proteins GLUT-1 and GLUT-5, and is phosphorylated by hexokinases to glucose-6-phosphate, which is trapped within the malignant cells. It is the increased glycolysis in cancer cells that is directly associated with the accumulation in PET imaging. FDG is most effectively trapped by tumors with slow or absent dephosphorylation, because malignant lesions have a higher glycolytic rate than normal tissue.[1] Furthermore, FDG

accumulation is increased in tumor hypoxia through activation of the glycolytic pathway.[26]

In the detedction of bone metastases, it is supposed that FDG is directly accumulated on the tumor cells but not on the enclosing bone tissues (Fig. 1).[27] In an early study,[28] the impact of ^{18}F-FDG PET in the detection of bone metastases was compared with planar bone scintigraphy in 23 patients with breast cancer. Bone scintigraphy was more sensitive in a subgroup of osteoblastic bone metastases; nevertheless, ^{18}F-FDG PET was able to detect more bone metastases overall, because of its ability to detect bone marrow as well as osteolytic lesions. Furthermore, mean standardized uptake values (SUVs) were substantially higher in osteolytic lesions than in osteoblastic lesions (6.6 vs 0.95, respectively).

In a comparative study, Ohta and colleagues[29] compared the diagnostic accuracy of ^{18}F-FDG PET with that of bone scintigraphy in 51 patients with breast cancer. Both imaging modalities showed similar sensitivity of 78%, but higher specificity was detected by ^{18}F-FDG PET (98% vs 80%). In another study of 48 patients with breast cancer, Yang and colleagues[30] reported a sensitivity of 93% for bone scintigraphy and 95% for ^{18}F-FDG PET, with similar accuracy of 95% for both modalities. In a retrospective study of 119 patients newly diagnosed with locally advanced breast cancer, bone scintigraphy, ^{18}F-FDG PET, CT, and plain radiography were compared as part of staging protocols.[31] ^{18}F-FDG PET showed a sensitivity and specificity of 87% and 92%, respectively compared with 67% and 99% for bone scintigraphy. Uematsu and colleagues[32] compared ^{18}F-FDG PET and bone SPECT in 15 patients with breast cancer and with known bone metastases, who had 143 osteoblastic and 20 osteolytic lesions. In a lesion-based analysis, the sensitivity of SPECT was significantly higher than ^{18}F-FDG PET (85% vs 17%) with similar specificity of 99% and 100% for SPECT and PET, respectively. The higher sensitivity of SPECT may mainly be due to a prominent number of sclerotic lesions. In another study, ^{18}F-FDG PET showed a sensitivity of 100% in the detection of osteolytic lesions, compared with 70% for bone scintigraphy.[33]

The discrepancies between findings on ^{18}F-FDG PET compared with those on bone scintigraphy may be mainly be due to different mechanisms of uptake. FDG uptake is higher in osteolytic metastases, because of larger amounts of tumor cells with high glycolytic rate.[23,28] By contrast, sclerotic metastases contain a smaller amount of viable tumor cells and hence show less FDG uptake.[23,28] Moreover, ^{18}F-FDG PET has the potential to detect

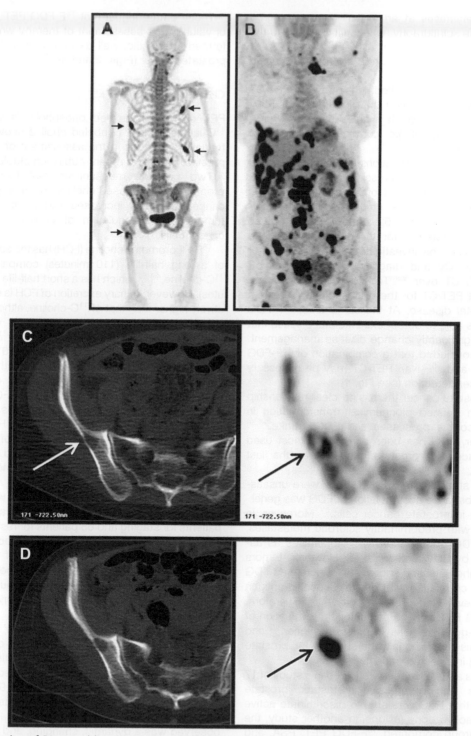

Fig. 1. Staging of 64-year-old patient with ovarian cancer (T3b N1 M1, FIGO 3C). (*A*) ^{18}F NaF PET (maximum intensity projection [MIP]) reveals multiple bone metastases on the skeleton (*arrows*). (*B*) ^{18}F-FDG PET MIP also reveals multiple metastases in the liver and retroperitoneum. (*C*) ^{18}F NaF PET/CT (transaxial slices): osteolytic lesion on the right ileum with NaF uptake only at the rim. (*D*) ^{18}F-FDG PET/CT (transaxial slices): osteolytic lesion on the right ileum with intense FDG uptake in the tumor cells.

bone metastases at an earlier stage compared with bone scintigraphy, when still confined to the bone marrow, before an osteoblastic pattern or reaction can be depicted by other imaging modalities.

In addition, the development of hybrid PET/CT scanners has improved the diagnostic accuracy of this modality, which enables metabolic function and morphologic correlation in a single acquisition.[19]

There are few publications that have compared [18]F NaF with either bone scintigraphy or ^{18}F-FDG PET in the assessment of bone metastases. In a recent prospective study, Iagaru and colleagues[34] examined 52 patients with proven malignancy referred for the evaluation of bone metastases. The investigators reported superior image quality and diagnostic accuracy of [18]F NaF PET/CT over ^{99m}Tc-MDP scintigraphy and ^{18}F-FDG PET/CT for the evaluation of the extent of skeletal disease. At the same time, ^{18}F-FDG PET was able to detect extraskeletal disease that could significantly change disease management. It was concluded that a combination of ^{18}F-FDG PET/CT and [18]F NaF PET/CT may be necessary for cancer detection (see **Fig. 1**).

In prostate cancer there is no clear relationship between defined biochemical transformation in the glycolysis processes and FDG uptake.[35,36] However, FDG has been one of the most used PET tracers in prostate cancer over the last decade.

Early studies with ^{18}F-FDG PET were unsatisfactory because accumulation of FDG was generally low in prostate cancer cells.[37] Moreover, in tumors with predominantly sclerotic metastases, lower FDG uptake than lytic metastases as assessed by SUV is seen.[28,38,39] However, tumors with higher Gleason scores show increased FDG uptake, correlating with prostate-specific antigen (PSA) level and PSA velocity.[40–42] Therefore, ^{18}F-FDG PET may be useful for the evaluation of tumor aggressiveness in prostate cancer,[40] and might also occasionally be suitable for prostate imaging in selected patients.[23,43–45]

Morris and colleagues[46] showed in a study of 17 patients with progressive metastatic prostate cancer that FDG was able to discriminate active from inactive bone lesions. In another study, the same group compared ^{18}F-FDG PET, PSA, and standard imaging in 22 patients undergoing chemotherapy for castration-resistance metastatic prostate cancer after 12 weeks of chemotherapy, and showed that in 94% of cases, PET correctly determined the clinical status of the patients. Disease progression was also correctly identified by ^{18}F-FDG PET in 91% of these cases.

These data suggest that ^{18}F-FDG PET may be of value in the assessment of therapy when performed at specific, well-defined clinical stages of prostate cancer (**Figs. 2** and **3**).[24]

CHOLINE DERIVATIVES

PET using radiolabeled phospholipids such as ^{11}C-labeled and ^{18}F-labeled choline showed potential advantages in the assessment of patients prostate cancer in recent published studies.[2–9]

Two possible mechanisms that have been proposed for increased choline uptake in prostate cancer cells are increased cell proliferation in tumors and upregulation of choline kinase in cancer cells.[47,48]

[18]F-Fluoromethylcholine (FCH) has the advantage of a long half-life (110 minutes) compared with ^{11}C-choline,[49–52] which has a short half-life (20 minutes). However, urinary excretion of FCH is comparatively higher than that of ^{11}C-choline, although this can be overcome by performing early dynamic imaging and using coregistered CT data.[53,54]

Cimitan and colleagues[2] examined 100 postoperative patients with prostate cancer with persistent raised serum PSA, suggestive of local recurrences or distant metastases. ^{18}F-FCH PET/CT correctly detected bone metastases in 21% of patients. In the authors' opinion, FCH uptake in bone seems to be highly predictive of skeletal metastases; however, this finding should be interpreted with caution in patients who are undergoing hormone therapy.[55]

In another study, ^{18}F-FCH PET/CT was performed on 111 patients with prostate cancer: 43 patients for staging and 68 patients for restaging.[56] The investigators found pathologic FCH accumulation in the skeleton in 15% (17/111) of patients, which was subsequently confirmed by bone scan, MRI, and CT morphology. It was concluded that ^{18}F-FCH PET/CT is well able to depict bone metastases in patients with prostate cancer.

In a prospective study by the authors' group,[57] the capability of ^{18}F-FCH PET/CT in the detection of bone marrow was examined in 70 patients with prostate cancer. ^{18}F-FCH PET/CT showed a sensitivity, specificity, and accuracy of 79%, 97%, and 84% for the detection of bone metastases in patients with prostate cancer (**Fig. 4**). Also observed was a dynamic, changing, and progressive pattern of abnormality associated with bone metastases: beginning with bone marrow involvement (without morphologic changes) then generally osteoblastic, but sometimes osteoclastic, changes (positive functional and morphologic findings), finally progressing to densely sclerotic lesions without any metabolic activity. In addition,

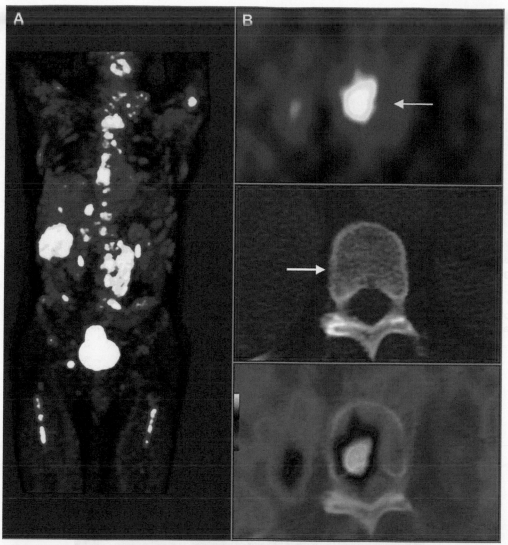

Fig. 2. ¹⁸F-FDG PET/CT in a patient with high-risk progressive prostate cancer. (*A*) ¹⁸F-FDG PET (MIP) shows multiple metastases (skeleton, liver; retroperitoneal lymph nodes). (*B*) Transaxial slices show bone marrow metastases (*yellow arrow*) without any morphologic changes on CT (*white arrow*).

¹⁸F-FCH PET/CT has shown promising results for the early detection of bone metastases when it is still confined to the medullary bone. Furthermore, the authors have found that a Hounsfield Units level of above 825 is associated with an absence of metabolic activity with FCH. Almost all of the FCH-negative sclerotic lesions were detected in patients who were undergoing hormone therapy, and this raises the possibility that these lesions may no longer be viable. Further clarification of such densely sclerotic but metabolically negative lesions is needed.

Using dual-time imaging, a significant increase of FCH uptake was seen in metastatic bone lesions on the late images (ie, 90 minutes postinjection). This finding confirmed the previous data reported by the authors' group[55,58,59] as well as those of other similar studies.[2,56] Another comparative study by the authors' group[60] attempted to determine the potential of ¹⁸F NaF PET/CT and ¹⁸F-FCH PET/CT for detecting bone metastases in 38 patients with prostate cancer. In a lesion-based analysis, the sensitivity and specificity of PET/CT in detection of bone metastasis were 81% and 93% by ¹⁸F NaF PET/CT and 74% and 99% by ¹⁸F-FCH PET/CT, respectively. In a patient-based analysis, there was good agreement between ¹⁸F-FCH and ¹⁸F NaF PET/CT ($\kappa = 0.76$).

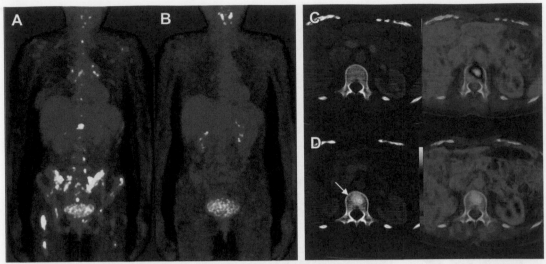

Fig. 3. ^{18}F-FDG PET/CT in a patient with breast cancer. (*A*) MIP image shows multiple bone metastases in the skeleton. (*B*) Follow-up study after therapy shows complete metabolic remission. (*C*) Primary staging: transaxial CT (*left*) and PET/CT fusion (*right*) slices of the thoracic spine show a solitary bone marrow metastasis without morphologic changes on CT. (*D*) Follow-up study: transaxial CT (*left*) and PET/CT fusion (*right*) slices of the thoracic spine no longer show metabolic activity on the sclerotic lesion seen on CT (*white arrow*).

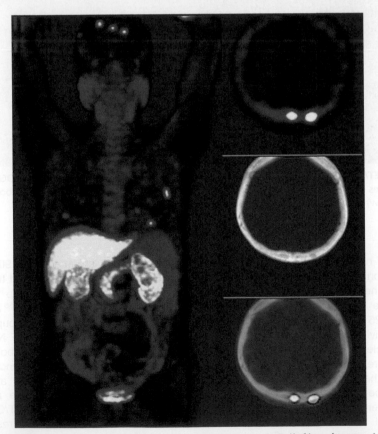

Fig. 4. ^{18}F-Choline PET/CT in restaging of a patient with prostate cancer. MIP (*left*) and transaxial slices of the skull (*right*) show multiple bone metastases (skull, ribs, vertebral spine).

[18]F NaF PET/CT demonstrated higher sensitivity than ^{18}F-FCH PET/CT in the detection of bone metastases, albeit not statistically significant.

^{18}F-FCH PET/CT has proved to be a more specific method than [18]F NaF PET/CT and has the potential for initial assessment of high-risk patients with prostate cancer, in particular for the early detection of bone marrow metastases. However, based on current knowledge, in patients with FCH-negative suspicious sclerotic lesions a second bone-seeking agent (eg, [18]F NaF) is recommended.

This study also showed that hormone therapy may be associated with increasing bone mineralization and sclerosis in malignant lesions, and that because of such a response to therapy, [18]F NaF PET could also be negative in highly dense sclerotic lesions. The authors also predict that [18]F NaF PET/CT will replace conventional bone imaging with ^{99m}Tc-labeled diphosphonates within the next few years.[23,24,61]

In a recent prospective study of 130 intermediate-risk and high-risk patients with prostate cancer, the therapy management was changed in 13 (10%) patients, mainly because of detection of bone metastases by ^{18}F-choline PET/CT; 2 patients had bone marrow metastases only detectable on choline PET studies.[62]

In a more recent study, Picchio and colleagues[63] compared the impact of ^{11}C-choline PET/CT with that of bone scintigraphy in 78 consecutive patients with biochemical progression of prostate cancer after primary treatment. The results of this study showed equivocal findings in 1 of 78 (1%) cases in ^{11}C-choline PET/CT and in 21 of 78 (27%) cases in bone scintigraphy. The ranges of sensitivity, specificity, positive predictive value, negative predictive value, and accuracy for ^{11}C-choline PET/CT were 89% to 89%, 98% to 100%, 96% to 100%, 94% to 96% and 95% to 96%, respectively depending on their attribution as either positive or negative. For bone scintigraphy these ranges were 100% to 70%, 75% to 100%, 68% to 100%, 100% to 86% and 83% to 90%, respectively. Concordant findings between ^{11}C-choline PET/CT and bone scintigraphy occurred in 55 of 78 (71%) cases. The accuracy of ^{11}C-choline PET/CT did not significantly differ between hormone-resistant patients (97%) and those who did not receive anti-androgenic treatment (95%). The investigators concluded that in clinical practice, ^{11}C-choline PET/CT may not replace bone scintigraphy because of its lower sensitivity. However, for its high specificity, positive findings on ^{11}C-choline PET/CT may accurately predict the presence of bone metastases. However, in the authors' opinion,[23,24] choline PET/CT is not only able to detect bone-marrow metastases but also provides important information concerning local recurrences as well as lymph node metastases, and has the potential to be a one-stop diagnostic procedure in the assessment of patients with prostate cancer and with biochemical evidence of recurrences.[64] Nevertheless, its prognostic value and cost-effectiveness compared with other imaging modalities are open issues that warrant evaluation in future studies.[64]

ACETATE DERIVATIVES

Many theories have been introduced for the mechanism of acetate accumulation in malignant cells, but the exact mechanism remains unclear. One approach to the molecular imaging of prostate cancer is to depict the malignant transformation of specific citrate metabolism of prostate epithelial cells.[65] The normal human prostate gland produces, accumulates, and secretes extraordinarily high levels of citrate. This is a unique capability, which does not exist in any other soft-tissue cells of the body. Malignant prostate epithelial cells undergo a metabolic transformation from citrate-producing normal cells to citrate-oxidizing malignant cells, leading to an increased turnover of acetate in prostate cancer. However, Yoshimoto and colleagues[66] suggest that acetate is incorporated into the lipid pool in cancer tissue with low oxidative metabolism and high lipid synthesis.

[11]C-Acetate has also been used for the imaging of prostate cancer during the last few years, and shows preferable characteristics for visualizing the pelvis because of its lack of urinary excretion and its acceptable tumor-to-background contrast.[41,67–70] Shreve and colleagues[68] suggested that ^{11}C-acetate has potential as a suitable tracer for imaging the genitourinary system.

The value of ^{11}C-acetate PET in the detection of prostate cancer recurrence has been assessed in some studies,[69,70] which reported a low sensitivity and discouraging results in postoperative patients especially in the case of PSA values less than 3 ng/mL.[69] Nevertheless, recent published data show that it might have significant potential for the detection of recurrences and metastases[71] when using more advanced PET/CT equipment.

More recently, ^{18}F-fluoroacetate has been introduced as a possible alternative to ^{11}C-acetate for PET imaging of prostate cancer, especially with respect to its longer half-life.[72,73]

In a recent pilot study[74] the feasibility of ^{11}C-acetate PET was compared with that of ^{18}F-FDG PET in the assessment of therapy response in patients with prostate cancer with known bone metastases. The results showed that ^{11}C-acetate

PET holds promise for the assessment of therapy response in prostate cancer bone metastases, and is complementary to ^{18}F-FDG PET in the detection of bone metastases.

[11]C-METHIONINE

The accumulation of ^{11}C-methionine in tumor cells is related to increased amino acid transport and protein synthesis.[75,76] Uptake of ^{11}C-methionine may reflect active tumor proliferation. However, few studies have investigated prostate cancer using ^{11}C-methionine PET.[10,11]

Nunez and colleagues[10] compared ^{11}C-methionine with ^{18}F-FDG PET in 12 patients with metastatic prostate cancer. The investigators reported that ^{11}C-methionine PET was more effective than ^{18}F-FDG PET for detecting bone metastases in this patient population. ^{11}C-methionine PET was able to detect 69.8% of metastatic bone lesions, in comparison with 48.3% for ^{18}F-FDG PET. The investigators supposed that the increased sensitivity of ^{11}C-methionine compared with ^{18}F-FDG PET may be the result of differences in tumor metabolism between patients, or a time-dependent metabolic cascade in metastatic prostate cancer, with initial uptake of ^{11}C-methionine in inactive lesions followed by increased uptake of FDG during progression of the disease.

In a recent retrospective study, Goudarzi and colleagues[77] evaluated the ability of diffusion-weighted imaging (DWI) to detect bone metastasis in 19 patients by comparing the results obtained using this modality with those obtained using ^{11}C-methionine PET and bone scintigraphy. The investigators reported that among 19 patients who were diagnosed using DWI and ^{11}C-methionine PET, ^{11}C-methionine PET identified 39 bone metastases, whereas DWI identified 60 malignant bony lesions out of 69 metastases revealed with conventional MRI. Among the 15 patients who were diagnosed using DWI and bone scintigraphy, bone scintigraphy identified 18 bone metastases, whereas DWI identified 72 of 78 metastases revealed with conventional MRI.

The overall bone metastasis detection rates were 56.5% for ^{11}C-methionine PET, 23.1% for bone scintigraphy, and 92.3% for DWI.

^{18}F-FLUORO-5α-DIHYDROTESTOSTERONE

A new imaging agent that binds to androgen receptors, ^{18}F-fluoro-5α-dihydrotestosterone (FDHT), has recently been developed.[12] FDHT, an androgen analogue, has been shown to accumulate in the prostate gland of nonhuman primates. The androgen receptor is highly functional and plays a major role in tumor growth despite the absence of its ligand dihydrotestosterone, even in castrated patients.[78,79]

In addition to conventional imaging methods, Larson and colleagues[80] used ^{18}F-FDG PET and ^{18}F-FDHT PET scans to examine 7 patients with progressive clinically metastatic prostate cancer. The investigators studied 59 lesions (10 soft-tissue lesions and 49 bone lesions) seen on standard imaging modalities. ^{18}F-FDG PET was positive in 57 of 59 lesions (97%) whereas ^{18}F-FDHT PET was positive in 46 of 59 lesions (78%).

In another study, Dehdashti and colleagues[81] evaluated the feasibility of using ^{18}F-FDHT PET in 19 patients with metastatic prostate cancer. ^{18}F-FDHT PET had a sensitivity of 63% and a lesion detection rate of 86% in a patient-based analysis. The study demonstrated a definite reduction in FDHT uptake in all lesions after patients had been treated acutely with an antiandrogen drug. The investigators concluded that tumor uptake of FDHT is a receptor-mediated process and that positive PET studies are associated with higher PSA levels. ^{18}F-FDHT PET shows promise in the analysis of antigen receptors and their impact on the clinical management of prostate cancer. ^{18}F-FDHT may also be a sensitive agent in the evaluation of therapy response.

^{18}F-FLUOROESTRADIOL

Estrogen as a steroidal hormone causes many physiologic effects, in particular by regulating gene expression by binding to specific estrogen receptors (ERs).[13] Estradiol, the most active form of estrogen in the human body, binds the ERs found in the cell nucleus of the female reproductive tract, breast, pituitary, hypothalamus, bone, liver, and other tissues.[82] Two types, αER and βER, have been described.[83] The specific binding of radiolabeled estradiol to the αER target was first reported by Jensen and colleagues.[84] Estradiol derivatives are lipophilic, transported via blood circulation, and are bound either to sex hormone–binding protein or to albumin. Binding of sex hormone protein keeps steroids from liver metabolism and assures their transport to target tissues.[13] Sex hormone–binding protein receptors are present in a higher percentage of ER-positive tumors (75%) than ER-negative tumors (37%).[13] Therefore, membrane sequestration of estradiol is supposed to particularly occur in hormone-responsive tumors.[13]

In the last 25 years, more than 20 fluorinated estrogen derivatives have been proposed for imaging purposes. 6α-^{18}F-fluoro-17β-estradiol (^{18}F-FES) is the most promising radiolabeled estrogen analogue, which shows a good ER-binding affinity and can be prepared for highly effective specific activity.[85,86] In the earliest reported ^{18}F-FES PET study,[87] an excellent correlation was found between FES uptake in the primary tumor measured on PET examination and the tumor ER concentration assessed in vitro by radioligand binding after surgery in 13 patients with primary breast cancer. In this study, ^{18}F-FES PET showed a sensitivity of 93% for the detection of metastatic lesions.

In a recent study by van Kruchten and colleagues,[88] ^{18}F-FES PET was performed in 33 patients with breast cancer presenting with a clinical dilemma, to determine its indication, diagnostic value, and therapeutic consequences in comparison with conventional imaging modalities. ^{18}F-FES PET was requested to evaluate equivocal lesions on conventional workup (n = 21), ER status in metastatic patients (n = 10), and the origin of metastases (n = 2). Twenty-two patients showed positive lesions on ^{18}F-FES PET. ^{18}F-FES PET was superior to conventional imaging, in particular for the assessment of bone metastases, detecting 341 bone lesions compared with 246 by conventional imaging. ^{18}F-FES PET improved diagnostic understanding in 88% of the patients and led to a change of therapy for 48 of the patients. The investigators concluded that with the exception of liver metastases, whole-body imaging of ER expression with ^{18}F-FES PET can be a valuable additional diagnostic tool when standard workup is inconclusive in patients with breast cancer.

SUMMARY

Bone imaging is performed for staging of disease, assessment of therapy, and detection of bone complications in patients with cancer. Assessment of bone metastases by imaging modalities is indicated for patients at high risk of bone involvement based on clinical findings.

Recently, PET/CT imaging has shown promising results for the assessment of bone metastases in patients with cancer. An unprecedented number of PET tracers have been tested for the assessment of malignant bone disease.

Specific PET tracers such as ^{18}F-FDG, ^{11}C-choline, and ^{18}F-choline show promising results, particularly in the early detection of metastatic bone disease and therapy monitoring, but inconsistent findings have been noted in densely sclerotic bone lesions, especially after therapy.

[18]F NaF PET demonstrates higher sensitivity than ^{18}F-FDG PET and ^{18}F-FCH PET for detection of bone metastases. However, ^{18}F-FDG PET and ^{18}F-FCH PET have shown the potential to be more specific methods than [18]F NaF PET, and have the potential to become one-stop diagnostic procedures for detecting both bone and soft-tissue disease, in particular for the early detection of bone marrow metastases.

In patients with suspicious sclerotic lesions but negative ^{18}F-FCH and ^{18}F-FDG PET, a second bone-seeking agent (eg, [18]F NaF) is suggested.

The question as to whether negative metabolic imaging in CT-positive bone metastases has any clinical relevance still remains, and is an issue that should challenge further studies.

Overall there are insufficient data available about other PET tracers such as acetate derivatives, ^{11}C-methionine, ^{18}F-FDHT, and ^{18}F-FES to draw conclusions concerning their potential value in the assessment of bone metastases.

REFERENCES

1. Warburg O. On the origin of cancer cells. Science 1956;123(3191):309–14.
2. Cimitan M, Bortolus R, Morassut S, et al. [(18)F]fluorocholine PET/CT imaging for the detection of recurrent prostate cancer at PSA relapse: experience in 100 consecutive patients. Eur J Nucl Med Mol Imaging 2006;33(12):1387–98.
3. Kwee SA, Wei H, Sesterhenn I, et al. Localization of primary prostate cancer with dual-phase ^{18}F-fluorocholine PET. J Nucl Med 2006;47(2):262–9.
4. Reske SN, Blumstein NM, Neumaier B, et al. Imaging prostate cancer with ^{11}C-choline PET/CT. J Nucl Med 2006;47(8):1249–54.
5. Hara T, Kosaka N, Shinoura N, et al. PET imaging of brain tumor with [methyl-^{11}C]choline. J Nucl Med 1997;38(6):842–7.
6. Hara T, Kosaka N, Kishi H. PET imaging of prostate cancer using carbon-11-choline. J Nucl Med 1998; 39(6):990–5.
7. Hara T, Inagaki K, Kosaka N, et al. Sensitive detection of mediastinal lymph node metastasis of lung cancer with ^{11}C-choline PET. J Nucl Med 2000; 41(9):1507–13.
8. Kobori O, Kirihara Y, Kosaka N, et al. Positron emission tomography of esophageal carcinoma using (11)C-choline and (18)F-fluorodeoxyglucose: a novel method of preoperative lymph node staging. Cancer 1999;86(9):1638–48.
9. Bauman G, Belhocine T, Kovacs M, et al. (18)F-fluorocholine for prostate cancer imaging: a systematic review of the literature. Prostate Cancer Prostatic Dis 2012;15(1):45–55.
10. Nunez R, Macapinlac HA, Yeung HW, et al. Combined ^{18}F-FDG and ^{11}C-methionine PET scans in patients with newly progressive metastatic prostate cancer. J Nucl Med 2002;43(1):46–55.
11. Toth G, Lengyel Z, Balkay L, et al. Detection of prostate cancer with ^{11}C-methionine positron emission tomography. J Urol 2005;173(1):66–9 [discussion: 69].

12. Bonasera TA, O'Neil JP, Xu M, et al. Preclinical evaluation of fluorine-18-labeled androgen receptor ligands in baboons. J Nucl Med 1996;37(6):1009–15.

13. Vallabhajosula S. (18)F-labeled positron emission tomographic radiopharmaceuticals in oncology: an overview of radiochemistry and mechanisms of tumor localization. Semin Nucl Med 2007;37(6):400–19.

14. Coleman RE. Skeletal complications of malignancy. Cancer 1997;80(Suppl 8):1588–94.

15. Berenson JR, Rajdev L, Broder M. Pathophysiology of bone metastases. Cancer Biol Ther 2006;5(9):1078–81.

16. Jemal A, Siegel R, Ward E, et al. Cancer statistics, 2007. CA Cancer J Clin 2007;57(1):43–66.

17. Blau M, Nagler W, Bender MA. Fluorine-18: a new isotope for bone scanning. J Nucl Med 1962;3:332–4.

18. Schirrmeister H, Guhlmann A, Elsner K, et al. Sensitivity in detecting osseous lesions depends on anatomic localization: planar bone scintigraphy versus ^{18}F PET. J Nucl Med 1999;40(10):1623–9.

19. Fogelman I, Cook G, Israel O, et al. Positron emission tomography and bone metastases. Semin Nucl Med 2005;35(2):135–42.

20. Petren-Mallmin M, Andreasson I, Ljunggren O, et al. Skeletal metastases from breast cancer: uptake of ^{18}F-fluoride measured with positron emission tomography in correlation with CT. Skeletal Radiol 1998;27(2):72–6.

21. Hawkins RA, Choi Y, Huang SC, et al. Evaluation of the skeletal kinetics of fluorine-18-fluoride ion with PET. J Nucl Med 1992;33(5):633–42.

22. Schirrmeister H, Guhlmann A, Kotzerke J, et al. Early detection and accurate description of extent of metastatic bone disease in breast cancer with fluoride ion and positron emission tomography. J Clin Oncol 1999;17(8):2381–9.

23. Langsteger W, Heinisch M, Fogelman I. The role of fluorodeoxyglucose, ^{18}F-dihydroxyphenylalanine, ^{18}F-choline, and ^{18}F-fluoride in bone imaging with emphasis on prostate and breast. Semin Nucl Med 2006;36(1):73–92.

24. Beheshti M, Langsteger W, Fogelman I. Prostate cancer: role of SPECT and PET in imaging bone metastases. Semin Nucl Med 2009;39(6):396–407.

25. Schirrmeister H. Detection of bone metastases in breast cancer by positron emission tomography. Radiol Clin North Am 2007;45(4):669–76, vi.

26. Minn H, Clavo AC, Wahl RL. Influence of hypoxia on tracer accumulation in squamous-cell carcinoma: in vitro evaluation for PET imaging. Nucl Med Biol 1996;23(8):941–6.

27. Ben-Haim S, Israel O. Breast cancer: role of SPECT and PET in imaging bone metastases. Semin Nucl Med 2009;39(6):408–15.

28. Cook GJ, Houston S, Rubens R, et al. Detection of bone metastases in breast cancer by [18]FDG PET: differing metabolic activity in osteoblastic and osteolytic lesions. J Clin Oncol 1998;16(10):3375–9.

29. Ohta M, Tokuda Y, Suzuki Y, et al. Whole body PET for the evaluation of bony metastases in patients with breast cancer: comparison with 99Tcm-MDP bone scintigraphy. Nucl Med Commun 2001;22(8):875–9.

30. Yang SN, Liang JA, Lin FJ, et al. Comparing whole body (18)F-2-deoxyglucose positron emission tomography and technetium-99m methylene diphosphonate bone scan to detect bone metastases in patients with breast cancer. J Cancer Res Clin Oncol 2002;128(6):325–8.

31. Mahner S, Schirrmacher S, Brenner W, et al. Comparison between positron emission tomography using 2-[fluorine-18]fluoro-2-deoxy-D-glucose, conventional imaging and computed tomography for staging of breast cancer. Ann Oncol 2008;19(7):1249–54.

32. Uematsu T, Yuen S, Yukisawa S, et al. Comparison of FDG PET and SPECT for detection of bone metastases in breast cancer. AJR Am J Roentgenol 2005;184(4):1266–73.

33. Nakai T, Okuyama C, Kubota T, et al. Pitfalls of FDG-PET for the diagnosis of osteoblastic bone metastases in patients with breast cancer. Eur J Nucl Med Mol Imaging 2005;32(11):1253–8.

34. Iagaru A, Mittra E, Dick DW, et al. Prospective evaluation of (99m)Tc MDP scintigraphy, (18)F NaF PET/CT, and (18)F FDG PET/CT for detection of skeletal metastases. Mol Imaging Biol 2012;14(2):252–9.

35. Singh G, Lakkis CL, Laucirica R, et al. Regulation of prostate cancer cell division by glucose. J Cell Physiol 1999;180(3):431–8.

36. Rossi F, Grzeskowiak M, Della Bianca V, et al. De novo synthesis of diacylglycerol from glucose. A new pathway of signal transduction in human neutrophils stimulated during phagocytosis of beta-glucan particles. J Biol Chem 1991;266(13):8034–8.

37. Effert PJ, Bares R, Handt S, et al. Metabolic imaging of untreated prostate cancer by positron emission tomography with 18fluorine-labeled deoxyglucose. J Urol 1996;155(3):994–8.

38. Shreve PD, Grossman HB, Gross MD, et al. Metastatic prostate cancer: initial findings of PET with 2-deoxy-2-[^{18}F]fluoro-D-glucose. Radiology 1996;199(3):751–6.

39. Yeh SD, Imbriaco M, Larson SM, et al. Detection of bony metastases of androgen-independent prostate cancer by PET-FDG. Nucl Med Biol 1996;23(6):693–7.

40. Seltzer MA, Barbaric Z, Belldegrun A, et al. Comparison of helical computerized tomography, positron emission tomography and monoclonal antibody scans for evaluation of lymph node metastases in patients with prostate specific antigen relapse after treatment for localized prostate cancer. J Urol 1999;162(4):1322–8.

41. Oyama N, Akino H, Kanamaru H, et al. ^{11}C-acetate PET imaging of prostate cancer. J Nucl Med 2002;43(2):181–6.

42. Agus DB, Golde DW, Sgouros G, et al. Positron emission tomography of a human prostate cancer xenograft: association of changes in deoxyglucose accumulation with other measures of outcome following androgen withdrawal. Cancer Res 1998; 58(14):3009–14.

43. Steinborn MM, Heuck AF, Tiling R, et al. Whole-body bone marrow MRI in patients with metastatic disease to the skeletal system. J Comput Assist Tomogr 1999;23(1):123–9.

44. Hetzel M, Hetzel J, Arslandemir C, et al. Reliability of symptoms to determine use of bone scans to identify bone metastases in lung cancer: prospective study. BMJ 2004;328(7447):1051–2.

45. Schirrmeister H, Arslandemir C, Glatting G, et al. Omission of bone scanning according to staging guidelines leads to futile therapy in non-small cell lung cancer. Eur J Nucl Med Mol Imaging 2004; 31(7):964–8.

46. Morris MJ, Akhurst T, Osman I, et al. Fluorinated deoxyglucose positron emission tomography imaging in progressive metastatic prostate cancer. Urology 2002;59(6):913–8.

47. Breeuwsma AJ, Pruim J, Jongen MM, et al. In vivo uptake of [^{11}C]choline does not correlate with cell proliferation in human prostate cancer. Eur J Nucl Med Mol Imaging 2005;32(6):668–73.

48. Zheng QH, Gardner TA, Raikwar S, et al. [^{11}C] Choline as a PET biomarker for assessment of prostate cancer tumor models. Bioorg Med Chem 2004; 12(11):2887–93.

49. Hara T, Kosaka N, Kishi H. Development of (18)F-fluoroethylcholine for cancer imaging with PET: synthesis, biochemistry, and prostate cancer imaging. J Nucl Med 2002;43(2):187–99.

50. DeGrado TR, Coleman RE, Wang S, et al. Synthesis and evaluation of ^{18}F-labeled choline as an oncologic tracer for positron emission tomography: initial findings in prostate cancer. Cancer Res 2001;61(1): 110–7.

51. DeGrado TR, Baldwin SW, Wang S, et al. Synthesis and evaluation of (18)F-labeled choline analogs as oncologic PET tracers. J Nucl Med 2001;42(12):1805–14.

52. DeGrado TR, Reiman RE, Price DT, et al. Pharmacokinetics and radiation dosimetry of ^{18}F-fluorocholine. J Nucl Med 2002;43(1):92–6.

53. Langsteger W, Beheshti M, Nader M, et al. Evaluation of lymph node and bone metastases with Fluor Choline (FCH) PET-CT in the follow up of prostate cancer patients. Eur J Nucl Med Mol Imaging 2006;33(Suppl 2):209.

54. Langsteger W, Beheshti M, Loidl W, et al. Fluor Choline (FCH) PET-CT in preoperative staging of prostate cancer. Eur J Nucl Med Mol Imaging 2006;33(Suppl 2):207–8.

55. Beheshti M, Vali R, Langsteger W. [^{18}F]fluorocholine PET/CT in the assessment of bone metastases in prostate cancer. Eur J Nucl Med Mol Imaging 2007;34(8):1316–7 [author reply: 1318–9].

56. Husarik DB, Miralbell R, Dubs M, et al. Evaluation of [(18)F]-choline PET/CT for staging and restaging of prostate cancer. Eur J Nucl Med Mol Imaging 2008;35(2):253–63.

57. Beheshti M, Vali R, Waldenberger P, et al. The use of ^{18}F choline PET in the assessment of bone metastases in prostate cancer: correlation with morphological changes on CT. Mol Imaging Biol 2009;11(6):446–54.

58. Langsteger W, Beheshti M, Pöcher S, et al. Fluor Choline (FCH) PET-CT in preoperative staging and follow up of prostate cancer. Mol Imaging Biol 2006;8:69.

59. Beheshti M, Haim S, Nader M, et al. Assessment of bone metastases in patients with prostate cancer by dual-phase F-18 Fluor Choline PET/CT. Eur J Nucl Med Mol I 2006;33(Suppl 2):208.

60. Beheshti M, Vali R, Waldenberger P, et al. Detection of bone metastases in patients with prostate cancer by ^{18}F fluorocholine and ^{18}F fluoride PET-CT: a comparative study. Eur J Nucl Med Mol Imaging 2008; 35(10):1766–74.

61. Alavi A, Kung JW, Zhuang H. Implications of PET based molecular imaging on the current and future practice of medicine. Semin Nucl Med 2004;34(1):56–69.

62. Beheshti M, Imamovic L, Broinger G, et al. ^{18}F choline PET/CT in the preoperative staging of prostate cancer in patients with intermediate or high risk of extracapsular disease: a prospective study of 130 patients. Radiology 2010;254(3): 925–33.

63. Picchio M, Spinapolice EG, Fallanca F, et al. [^{11}C] choline PET/CT detection of bone metastases in patients with PSA progression after primary treatment for prostate cancer: comparison with bone scintigraphy. Eur J Nucl Med Mol Imaging 2012; 39(1):13–26.

64. Beheshti M, Langsteger W. Choline PET/CT compared with bone scintigraphy in the detection of bone metastases in prostate cancer patients. Eur J Nucl Med Mol Imaging 2012;39(5):910–1.

65. Costello LC, Franklin RB. Citrate metabolism of normal and malignant prostate epithelial cells. Urology 1997;50(1):3–12.

66. Yoshimoto M, Waki A, Yonekura Y, et al. Characterization of acetate metabolism in tumor cells in relation to cell proliferation: acetate metabolism in tumor cells. Nucl Med Biol 2001;28(2):117–22.

67. Shreve PD, Gross MD. Imaging of the pancreas and related diseases with PET carbon-11-acetate. J Nucl Med 1997;38(8):1305–10.

68. Shreve P, Chiao PC, Humes HD, et al. Carbon-11-acetate PET imaging in renal disease. J Nucl Med 1995;36(9):1595–601.

69. Oyama N, Miller TR, Dehdashti F, et al. ^{11}C-acetate PET imaging of prostate cancer: detection of

recurrent disease at PSA relapse. J Nucl Med 2003; 44(4):549–55.

70. Kotzerke J, Volkmer BG, Neumaier B, et al. Carbon-11 acetate positron emission tomography can detect local recurrence of prostate cancer. Eur J Nucl Med Mol Imaging 2002;29(10):1380–4.

71. Albrecht S, Buchegger F, Soloviev D, et al. (11)C-acetate PET in the early evaluation of prostate cancer recurrence. Eur J Nucl Med Mol Imaging 2007;34(2):185–96.

72. Ponde DE, Dence CS, Oyama N, et al. ^{18}F-fluoroacetate: a potential acetate analog for prostate tumor imaging—in vivo evaluation of ^{18}F-fluoroacetate versus ^{11}C-acetate. J Nucl Med 2007;48(3):420–8.

73. Matthies A, Ezziddin S, Ulrich EM, et al. Imaging of prostate cancer metastases with ^{18}F-fluoroacetate using PET/CT. Eur J Nucl Med Mol Imaging 2004; 31(5):797.

74. Mitra AV, Bancroft EK, Barbachano Y, et al. Targeted prostate cancer screening in men with mutations in BRCA1 and BRCA2 detects aggressive prostate cancer: preliminary analysis of the results of the IMPACT study. BJU Int 2011;107(1):28–39.

75. Ishiwata K, Ido T, Vaalburg W. Increased amounts of D-enantiomer dependent on alkaline concentration in the synthesis of L-[methyl-^{11}C]methionine. Int J Rad Appl Instrum A 1988;39(4):311–4.

76. Miyazawa H, Arai T, Iio M, et al. PET imaging of non-small-cell lung carcinoma with carbon-11-methionine: relationship between radioactivity uptake and flow-cytometric parameters. J Nucl Med 1993;34(11): 1886–91.

77. Goudarzi B, Kishimoto R, Komatsu S, et al. Detection of bone metastases using diffusion weighted magnetic resonance imaging: comparison with (11)C-methionine PET and bone scintigraphy. Magn Reson Imaging 2010;28(3):372–9.

78. Apolo AB, Pandit-Taskar N, Morris MJ. Novel tracers and their development for the imaging of

metastatic prostate cancer. J Nucl Med 2008; 49(12):2031–41.

79. Scher HI, Sawyers CL. Biology of progressive, castration-resistant prostate cancer: directed therapies targeting the androgen-receptor signaling axis. J Clin Oncol 2005;23(32):8253–61.

80. Larson SM, Morris M, Gunther I, et al. Tumor localization of 16beta-^{18}F-fluoro-5alpha-dihydrotestosterone versus ^{18}F-FDG in patients with progressive, metastatic prostate cancer. J Nucl Med 2004; 45(3):366–73.

81. Dehdashti F, Picus J, Michalski JM, et al. Positron tomographic assessment of androgen receptors in prostatic carcinoma. Eur J Nucl Med Mol Imaging 2005;32(3):344–50.

82. Van de Wiele C, De Vos F, Slegers G, et al. Radiolabeled estradiol derivatives to predict response to hormonal treatment in breast cancer: a review. Eur J Nucl Med 2000;27(9):1421–33.

83. Mosselman S, Polman J, Dijkema R. ER beta: identification and characterization of a novel human estrogen receptor. FEBS Lett 1996;392(1):49–53.

84. Jensen EV, Desombre ER, Kawashima T, et al. Estrogen-binding substances of target tissues. Science 1967;158(3800):529–30.

85. Mankoff DA, Shields AF, Krohn KA. PET imaging of cellular proliferation. Radiol Clin North Am 2005; 43(1):153–67.

86. Kiesewetter DO, Kilbourn MR, Landvatter SW, et al. Preparation of four fluorine-18-labeled estrogens and their selective uptakes in target tissues of immature rats. J Nucl Med 1984;25(11):1212–21.

87. Mintun MA, Welch MJ, Siegel BA, et al. Breast cancer: PET imaging of estrogen receptors. Radiology 1988;169(1):45–8.

88. van Kruchten M, Glaudemans AW, de Vries EF, et al. PET imaging of estrogen receptors as a diagnostic tool for breast cancer patients presenting with a clinical dilemma. J Nucl Med 2012;53(2):182–90.

^{18}F NaF PET/CT and Conventional Bone Scanning in Routine Clinical Practice
Comparative Analysis of Tracers, Clinical Acquisition Protocols, and Performance Indices

Gad Abikhzer, MDCM, FRCPC, ABNM[a],[*],[1], John Kennedy, PhD[a], Ora Israel, MD[a],[b]

KEYWORDS

- Bone scan • F-18 fluoride • PET/CT • Whole body SPECT

KEY POINTS

- Conventional planar and SPECT bone scintigraphy is an established technique.
- F-18 fluoride PET/CT has the potential to become the gold standard in functional bone imaging.
- A thorough comparison of both techniques, including advantages and disadvantages are discussed.
- Future directions of both modalities are analyzed.

INTRODUCTION

Bone scintigraphy (BS) was one of the earliest examinations performed in nuclear medicine. F-18 sodium fluoride (NaF) is a bone-scanning agent that was first introduced in 1962.[1] The high 511 keV energy annihilation photons emitted by F-18 could be imaged at that time with rectilinear scanners equipped with thick crystals. For present day standards, the images obtained were of poor quality. With the advent of the first technetium-99m (Tc)-based phosphonates in 1971 followed by methylene disphosphonate (MDP)[2] and the development of the Anger camera, fluoride bone scanning was replaced. BS has become one of the most common procedures, widely used in the evaluation of malignant and benign diseases of the skeleton. The advent of single-photon emission tomography (SPECT) and eventually SPECT/computed tomography (CT) has further increased the diagnostic accuracy of BS and its clinical applications.[3] Over the past few years, with the rapidly increasing implementation of PET/CT devices and F-18, there has been a reemergence of interest and use of NaF.

There are now 2 excellent bone-scanning agents available, and the nuclear medicine community is faced with the dilemma of which one to adopt in routine clinical use. Tc-MDP has withstood the test of time, is easily available from generators even in remote locations, and can be used with the easily accessible gamma cameras that currently

The authors have nothing to disclose.
a Department of Nuclear Medicine, Rambam Health Care Campus, 6 Ha'Aliya Street, Haifa 31096, Israel; b B. and R. Rapaport Faculty of Medicine, Technion–Israel Institute of Technology, Haifa, Israel
1 Dr Abikhzer is a clinical and research fellow supported by the Azrieli foundation and the Dr Dov Front scholarship fund of the Rambam Health Care Campus R&D foundation.
* Corresponding author.
E-mail address: gad101@hotmail.com

PET Clin 7 (2012) 315–328
doi:10.1016/j.cpet.2012.04.005

outnumber PET/CT devices. On the other hand, PET/CT devices are becoming readily available worldwide, together with cyclotrons and distribution networks for ^{18}F-fluorodeoxyglucose (FDG), and this has facilitated as well the use of NaF in routine clinical work. Although there are a number of advantages to the use of NaF, which will be described in this article, do the excellent pharmacokinetic properties of this tracer and superior resolution of PET/CT devices translate to clinical benefits?

PHARMACOKINETICS AND UPTAKE MECHANISM

Comparison of the pharmacokinetics of Tc-MDP and NaF offer a theoretical advantage for NaF. First-pass clearance of Tc-based phosphonates is approximately 64%.[4] Protein binding of Tc-MDP is 25% to 30% immediately after injection and approximately 50% at 4 hours.[5] It does not bind to red blood cells (RBCs). Imaging with Tc-MDP requires a 2-hour to 4-hour uptake time after injection, when 40% of the tracer is found in skeleton, 40% in urine, 10% in soft tissues, and only 5% in the blood stream, which results in improved target-to-background ratio and better image quality.[2] NaF undergoes more rapid blood clearance, with first-pass clearance close to 100%,[6] as it has negligible protein binding. Approximately 30% of the injected dose is in RBCs, which does not interfere with bone uptake, as NaF freely diffuses across the cell membrane.[7] Plasma clearance is very rapid. Approximately 50% of the injected NaF is taken up in bone,[8] with the remainder excreted by the kidneys by 6 hours after tracer administration.[9] These properties permit a shorter uptake time of NaF with earlier start of imaging (Table 1).

Bone is composed of two-thirds mineral and one-third collagen, extracellular matrix, and a variety of bone-lining cells. The mineral matrix is composed of calcium hydroxyapatite, Ca10(OH)2(PO4)6, containing calcium phosphate that can be exchanged with phosphonates present in MDP.[2]

Tc-MDP uptake in bone is considered to be mainly related to chemisorption of the disphosphonate onto the surface of hydroxyapatite, followed by incorporation into the crystal. Bone uptake of Tc-MDP is related to increased blood flow and capillary permeability, as well as to increased bone turnover with osteoid formation. Uptake of Tc-MDP in immature collagen has also been described.[2] Uptake of NaF has a similar mechanism to Tc-MDP. Following chemisorption of fluoride ions onto the surface of hydroxyapatite, they exchange with the hydroxyl (OH$^-$) ions in the crystal, forming fluoroapatite.[4]

Imaging Protocols

Requisition and history
Requisition for BS and NaF PET/CT by the referring physician should ideally be accompanied by a concise summary of the patient's history with a pertinent clinical question. The following points are very important for accurate interpretation of the examination, depending on the clinical indication.

- History of malignancy
- Date of recent chemotherapy
- Previous fractures or recent trauma
- Previous orthopedic surgery and relevant dates
- Previous infection and its location
- Urinary diversion procedures
- Location of any bone pain.

Previous bone scintigraphy, as well as other relevant imaging studies, should be available for comparison.[10]

Patient preparation
The preparation of patients referred for BS and NaF PET/CT is essentially the same. Patients should be well hydrated before the study and during the uptake period between the time of tracer injection and imaging. This enhances renal excretion, resulting in improved target-to-background ratio and reducing radiation exposure of the patients. Patients are also encouraged to drink more frequently for the remainder of the day. Immediately before image acquisition, patients are asked to empty their bladders. Any metal objects should be removed to prevent attenuation artifacts.[10]

Radiopharmaceutical, injected activity, and uptake time
BS using Tc-MDP (other phosphonate-based tracers are also available, such as di-carboxy

---

Table 1
Comparison of pharmacokinetic properties of Tc-MDP and NaF

	MDP	NaF
Urinary excretion	70% after 6 h[4]	50% after 6 h[9]
Protein binding	50% at 4 h[5]	Negligible[7]
RBC binding	Negligible[5]	30%[7]
First-pass clearance	~64%[4]	Nearly 100%[6]
% bone uptake	35%–50%[2]	50%[8]

Abbreviations: MDP, methylene disphosphonate; NaF, sodium fluoride; Tc, technetium.

propane-diphosphonate [DPD] and hydroxy-methylene disphosphonate [HDP]):

- Adults: 740 to 1110 MBq (20–30 mCi) is injected intravenously (IV). The administered activity should be increased in obese patients to 11 to 13 MBq/kg (300–350 µCi/kg). Injection should be performed ideally with an IV catheter rather than through direct venipuncture, as injection site infiltrations can cause discomfort to the patient and result in reconstruction streak artifacts, most notably with SPECT.
- Pediatrics: 9 to 11 MBq/kg (250–300 µCi/kg) is administered with a minimum activity of 20 to 40 MBq (0.5–1.0 mCi) and maximum activity that should not exceed adult doses.[10]

Tc-MDP preparation uses simple, commercial kits, thus permitting greater department flexibility when additional studies are scheduled at the last minute or emergency BS is requested (**Table 2**).

PET/CT using NaF:

- Adults: 185 to 370 MBq (5–10 mCi) is injected IV, through a catheter. For obese patients, injected activity should be at the upper limit of recommended doses.
- Pediatrics: 2.59 MBq/kg, 70 µCi/kg is administered with a minimum activity of 11 MBq (0.3 mCi) and the maximum level not exceeding 185 MBq (5 mCi).[11]

The shorter half-life of NaF requires more rigid scheduling and lowers the ability to make unexpected changes in the clinical daily schedule (see **Table 2**).

Oral administration of NaF has been used previously. It appears to be as effective as IV administration, as the intestinal absorption of NaF is prompt and complete. Residual NaF in the gastrointestinal tract may occasionally remain in certain patients with incomplete absorption.[12] With current PET/CT technology, this should not cause a diagnostic dilemma. This route of administration may represent an alternative to IV injection in patients with difficult venous access.

Although peak bone activity for Tc-MDP is 1 hour post injection, soft tissue clearance is nearly complete at 4 hours, with imaging generally performed at 2 to 4 hours post injection. NaF PET/CT is a more rapid overall examination. The uptake time is usually 30 to 45 minutes for patients with normal renal function. A 90-minute to 120-minute wait is recommended when imaging the lower extremities.[11]

Image acquisition

BS and SPECT BS acquisition protocols vary depending on the routine work flows in different departments. Standard planar scintigraphy is performed at 2 to 4 hours after injection. A 3-phase, or occasionally a 4-phase study, can be also performed. The flow (first phase) and blood pool (second phase) studies add important information to the standard BS (third phase). They assess the presence of blood flow abnormalities (increased perfusion is the more frequent finding) that may occur in various clinical settings, such as osteomyelitis, complex regional pain syndrome, and heterotopic ossifications, as well as in primary bone tumors, avascular necrosis, Paget disease, or fractures. The 24-hour delayed phase (fourth phase) improves bone-to–soft tissue differentiation and is therefore useful in the elderly, in patients with diabetes, or those with peripheral venous disease in whom increased transit and uptake time impair image quality, mainly of the lower extremities.[2] It can also be used when high amounts of the radiopharmaceutical retained in the urinary tract (eg, a full urinary bladder) obscure pelvic bone structures, or when urinary contamination is present on the 3-hour scan and is

Table 2
Comparison of administered dose, uptake time of radiopharmaceuticals, and radiation dosimetry of Tc-MDP and NaF

	Tc-99m MDP BS[1]	18F NaF PET/CT [11]
Dosage (adult)	740–1110 MBq (20–30 mCi)	185–370 MBq (5–10 mCi)
Dosage (pediatric)	9–11 MBq/kg (250–300 µCi/kg)	2.59 MBq/kg (70 µCi/kg)
Time to imaging	2–4 h	30–45 minutes (90–120 minutes for extremities)
Radiation dosimetry	4.2 mSv (planar BS) 7.4 mSv (SPECT/CT)	12.1 mSv

Abbreviations: BS, bone scintigraphy; CT, computed tomography; MDP, methylene disphosphonate; NaF, sodium fluoride; SPECT, single-photon emission computed tomography; Tc-99m, technetium-99m.

expected to disappear on delayed images. With the use of SPECT imaging, this phase is less often required.

SPECT imaging as an adjunct to BS improves contrast resolution, and enables better separation of adjacent structures and identification of lesions obscured by the 2-dimensional planar images. Sensitivity of BS has improved with SPECT, with 20% to 50% more vertebral lesions, for example, being detected than with planar BS only. Specificity of BS with SPECT is also higher because of more accurate lesion localization.[3]

Low-energy, high-resolution (LEHR) collimators are used for whole-body planar BS and SPECT. Flow/perfusion and blood pool scans aiming at detection of hyperemia are performed immediately after the injection of Tc-MDP, including a less than 1-minute dynamic study (eg, 16 frames at 2 seconds per frame), immediately followed by approximately 300 kcounts anterior and posterior planar scans (1024 × 256 matrix) of a specific region of interest. The planar whole-body scan is performed using continuous bed motion for 1500 kcounts with a 256 × 1024 matrix. A typical SPECT bone-acquisition protocol uses 2 detectors for 60 to 120 stops over a 360° scan with 10 to 40 seconds per stop. Reconstruction matrix is at least 64 × 64 (Table 3).[10]

With conventional gamma cameras, routine acquisition time for planar BS of the entire skeleton is approximately 12 minutes, followed by a single field-of-view (FOV) SPECT of about 15 minutes. SPECT acquisition time can be reduced by a factor of 2 while maintaining image quality[13] with the use of collimator-detector response compensation in image reconstruction, also known as resolution recovery. Iterative reconstruction is typically used and images are post-filtered to reduce noise. Available reconstruction software products include Wide Beam Reconstruction (UltraSPECT, Haifa,

Israel), Evolution (GE Healthcare, Waukesha, WI, USA), Astonish (Philips Healthcare, Best, Netherlands), and Flash 3D (Siemens Healthcare, Erlangen, Germany).

NaF PET To obtain high-quality skeletal images on current devices, emission scans with acquisition times of 1 to 2 minutes per bed position in 3-dimensional mode are obtained, depending on the camera, injected activity, uptake time, and body habitus of the patient. For a scan range from the skull to upper thighs with an average of 9 bed positions, acquisition time is in the range of 9 to 18 minutes, including CT acquisition and bed translation, longer for a whole body study, which requires an average of 15 bed positions. Reconstruction typically uses 3-dimensional maximum likelihood expectation maximization (MLEM) algorithm and a 128 × 128 or 256 × 256 matrix, with post filtering. A maximum intensity projection (MIP) image that is generated can facilitate detection of suspicious regions of interest for diagnosis (Fig. 1, Table 4).[11]

Dynamic studies for NaF PET studies have been performed for investigational purposes to provide quantitation of kinetic NaF incorporation parameters.[14,15]

Hybrid imaging of the bone Hybrid scanners provide the ability to perform emission and CT scans sequentially in a single imaging session on a single imaging device. For PET/CT, whole-body helical CT is acquired either immediately before or after the emission scan to provide CT-based attenuation correction and anatomic localization. Typical settings for an attenuation correction/localization CT scan are a tube current of 30 mA, voltage of 120 kVp, rotation of 0.5 second, and pitch of 1.[11] CT parameters can be modified, aiming at either reduced radiation exposure to the patient, associated with a poorer image quality, or alternatively, to provide diagnostic studies if required.

SPECT/CT is typically limited to a region of interest defined by suspicious findings in the skeleton detected on the planar component of the study, or guided by specific patient symptoms or previous findings. The duration of the CT acquisition depends on the type of CT component of the specific imaging device, ranging from 5 minutes for 1 bed position for a hybrid SPECT/CT with an x-ray tube mounted on the same gantry as the gamma camera detectors, to less than 1 minute for a hybrid PET or SPECT device with a multislice CT.

Radiation Dosimetry

The effective dose to the patient from an injection of 370 MBq of NaF is about 8.9 mSv compared

Table 3
Sample image acquisition protocol for BS

Collimator	LEHR
Flow	2 s/frame for a total of 32 seconds
Blood pool	~300 kcount anterior and posterior scans
Planar skeletal phase	1500 kcounts whole-body scan
SPECT	60–120 stops, over a 360° scan, 10–40 s per stop, 64 × 64 matrix reconstruction

Abbreviations: BS, bone scintigraphy; LEHR, low-energy, high-resolution; SPECT, single-photon emission computed tomography.

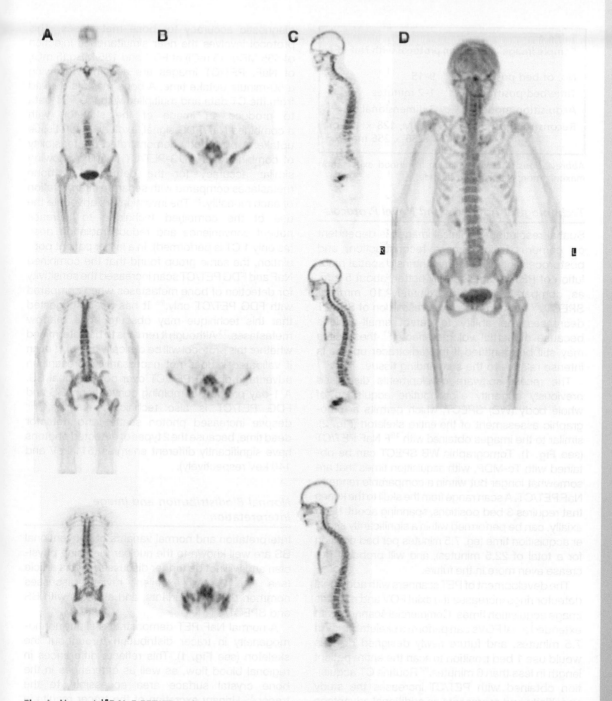

Fig. 1. Normal ^{18}F NaF PET/CT with coronal (*A*), axial (*B*), sagittal (*C*), and MIP (*D*) reconstructions. Note slightly heterogeneous bone tracer distribution throughout the skeleton.

with 4.2 mSv for 740 MBq of Tc-MDP for SPECT.[11] A meta-analysis reported a range of values of 2.7 to 15.0 mSv for NaF versus 4.2 to 5.7 mSv for Tc-MDP, respectively.[16] In children, these values are lower.[17] The radiation exposure associated with the CT component of PET/CT and SPECT/CT studies is highly variable and ranges from less than 1 mSv for CT-attenuation correction only,[18] to about 8 mSv for a diagnostic CT scan.[19] A typical value for an effective CT dose used for localization and attenuation correction is 3.2 mSv.[11] Consequently, the total effective dose of a NaF PET with a localization CT bone scan is approximately 12.1 mSv compared with approximately 7.4 mSv for a bone SPECT/CT (see **Table 2**).

Table 4
Sample image acquisition protocol with NaF PET

No. of bed positions	9–15
Time/bed position	1–2 minutes
Acquisition mode	3 dimensional
Reconstruction	MLEM, 128 × 128 or 256 × 256 matrix

Abbreviations: MLEM, maximum likelihood expectation maximization; NaF, sodium fluoride.

Technological Advances and Novel Protocols

Spatial resolution of clinical images is dependent on camera design, image reconstruction, and postprocessing. The current intrinsic spatial resolution of PET is considerably better, about 5 mm, as compared with approximately 10 mm for SPECT.[20] Although the lower resolution of SPECT decreases the ability to detect small lesions because of partial volume effects,[21] these sites may still be identified if the radiotracer uptake is intense relative to the surrounding tissue.

The recent software developments discussed previously currently allow routine acquisition of whole body (WB) SPECT, which permits a tomographic assessment of the entire skeleton (**Fig. 2**), similar to the images obtained with [18]F NaF PET/CT (see **Fig. 1**). Tomographic WB SPECT can be obtained with Tc-MDP, with acquisition times that are somewhat longer but within a comparable range to NaF PET/CT. A scan range from the skull to the knees that requires 3 bed positions, spanning about 1.2 m axially, can be performed within a significantly shorter acquisition time (eg, 7.5 minutes per bed position for a total of 22.5 minutes), and will probably decrease even more in the future.

The development of PET scanners with additional detector rings increases the axial FOV and reduces image acquisition times. Commercial scanners with extended axial FOVs can perform a skeletal study in 7.5 minutes, and future newly designed devices would use 1 bed position to scan the entire patient length in less than 6 minutes.[22] Routine CT acquisition obtained with PET/CT increases the study specificity and represents an additional advantage of NaF PET/CT compared with BS.[23]

WB PET/magnetic resonance (MR) imaging scanners have also been developed. WB MR imaging sequences are very accurate for the evaluation of bone and bone marrow metastases.[24] A hybrid PET/MR scan following the injection of NaF and/or FDG may represent in the future the 1-stop bone-imaging modality.

Sequential injection and imaging of FDG and NaF has been described, attempting to increase the diagnostic accuracy for bone metastases. This protocol involves the near simultaneous injection of 555 MBq (15 mCi) of FDG and 185 MBq (5 mCi) of NaF. PET/CT images are acquired following a 60-minute uptake time. A bone mask is derived from the CT data and multiplied with the PET data to produce an image of the skeleton with a combined NaF/FDG signal, excluding soft tissue uptake. A pilot study demonstrated the feasibility of combined NaF/FDG-PET/CT imaging showing similar accuracy for the detection of bone metastases compared with separate interpretation of each modality.[25] The investigators advocate the use of the combined technique to increase patient convenience and reduce radiation dose (as only 1 CT is performed). In a larger patient population, the same group found that the combined NaF and FDG PET/CT scan increased the sensitivity for detection of bone metastases when compared with FDG PET/CT only.[26] It has been suggested that this technique may obscure bone marrow metastases.[11] Although it remains to be determined whether this protocol will be clinically useful,[27] even if validated it does not necessarily represent an advantage of NaF PET/CT over conventional BS. A 1-day protocol combining conventional BS and FDG PET/CT is also technically feasible,[28,29] despite increased photon scatter and detector dead time, because the 2 types of detected photons have significantly different energies (511 keV and 140 keV respectively).

Normal Biodistribution and Image Interpretation

Interpretation and normal variants of conventional BS are well known to the nuclear medicine physician and will not be further discussed in this article (see **Fig. 2**). An excellent review discusses common patterns, variants, and artifacts with BS and SPECT/CT.[30]

A normal NaF PET demonstrates slight nonhomogeneity in tracer distribution throughout the skeleton (see **Fig. 1**). This reflects differences in regional blood flow, as well as differences in the bone crystal surface area accessible to the tracer.[12] Urinary excretion of the tracer results in kidney and urinary bladder visualization.

Interpretation of both types of bone scans is similar, with the same patterns of abnormal uptake to be expected (**Figs. 3** and **4**). Any causes of altered bone metabolism may cause increased NaF uptake (**Fig. 5**), which at present is most often used for metastatic disease (see **Fig. 3**). Uptake may be quite prominent in benign findings as well. NaF PET/CT has a high sensitivity for detecting lytic lesions (**Fig. 6**).[31] For those who are

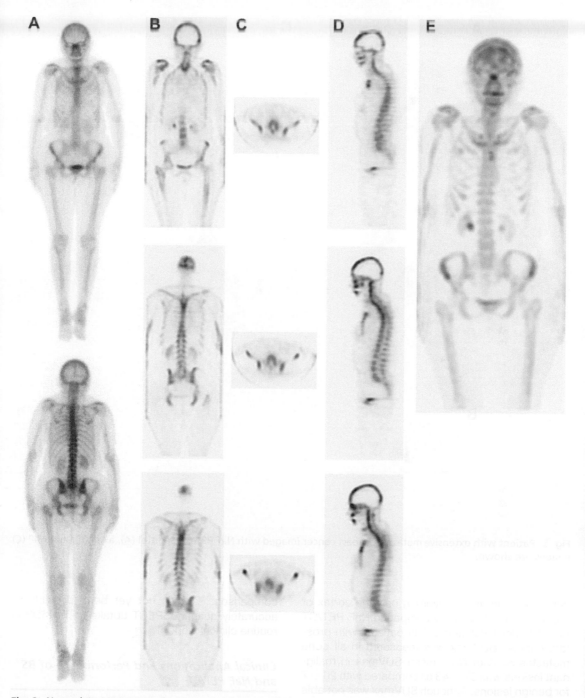

Fig. 2. Normal Tc-MDP BS in the same patient as in **Fig. 1**: Planar (*A*) and WB SPECT with coronal (*B*), axial (*C*), sagittal (*D*), and MIP (*E*) reconstructions.

routinely reading BS, a learning curve is associated with the interpretation of NaF PET/CT before becoming familiar with the normal and sometimes prominent heterogeneity of tracer distribution.

Only a few studies have assessed NaF standard uptake values (SUVs), which are not routinely used

in the interpretation of NaF PET/CT at present. One study measured the SUVmax of NaF uptake in metastatic lesions in a variety of malignancies. Sclerotic or mixed lesions had higher SUV values than lytic sites. The same was found for lesions involving both the cortex and medulla when

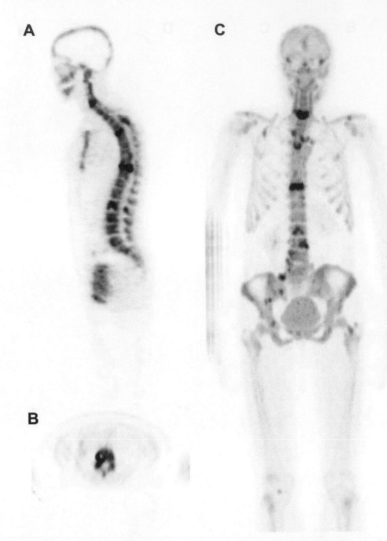

Fig. 3. Patient with extensive metastatic breast cancer imaged with NaF PET/CT. Sagittal (*A*), axial (*B*), and MIP (*C*) images are shown.

compared with those involving only the cortex or the medulla.[32] In a study comparing NaF PET/CT to F-18 fluorocholine (FCH) in patients with prostate cancer, SUVmax was measured in all bone metastases. With NaF, mean SUVmax in malignant lesions was 57 ± 43 as compared with 20 ± 7 for benign lesions. Although SUVmax was not able to differentiate between benign and malignant lesions, none of the benign lesions had an SUVmax higher than 45.[33] The applicability of this statement in routine clinical work is questionable, as certain benign bone entities, including fibrous dysplasia, Paget disease, and acute fractures, can demonstrate very intense uptake. Interval changes in SUVmax have been found in a few patients to be able to predict response to therapy, even in the absence of differences on visual

comparison.[34] It has not yet been possible to accurately quantify SPECT uptake of Tc-MDP in routine clinical work.[35]

Clinical Applications and Performance of BS and NaF PET/CT

This issue of the *PET Clinics* reviews the clinical utility of NaF PET in the assessment of a variety of bone diseases. Various clinical indications and potential applications for NaF PET/CT and/or BS are summarized in **Box 1** and are reviewed in depth in the appropriate articles.

To accurately assess both technologies, studies have to compare similar state-of-the-art technologies. This is analogous to the classic idiom of the need to compare apples with apples

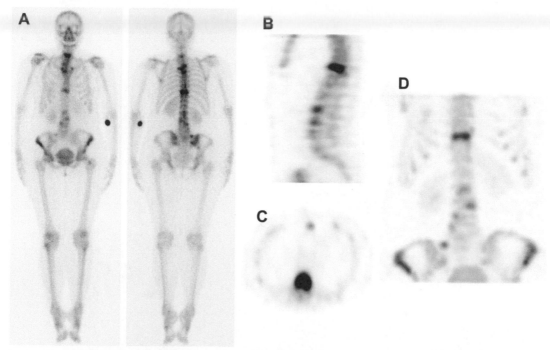

Fig. 4. Patient with extensive metastatic breast cancer imaged with Tc-MDP BS (same patient as in **Fig. 3**). Planar (A) and SPECT with sagittal (B), axial (C), and MIP (D) images are shown.

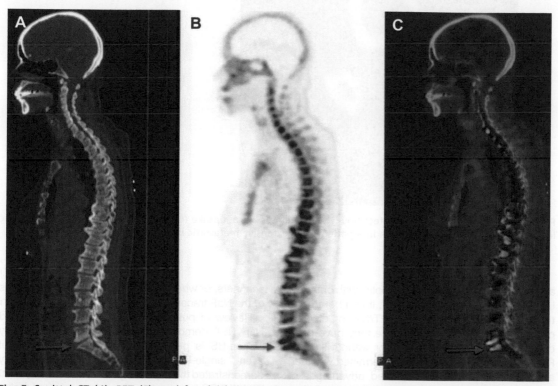

Fig. 5. Sagittal CT (A), PET (B), and fused (C) images from NaF PET/CT showing increased uptake in multiple osteophytes in the lower thoracic and upper lumbar spine and in L5/S1 degenerative disc disease (*arrow*).

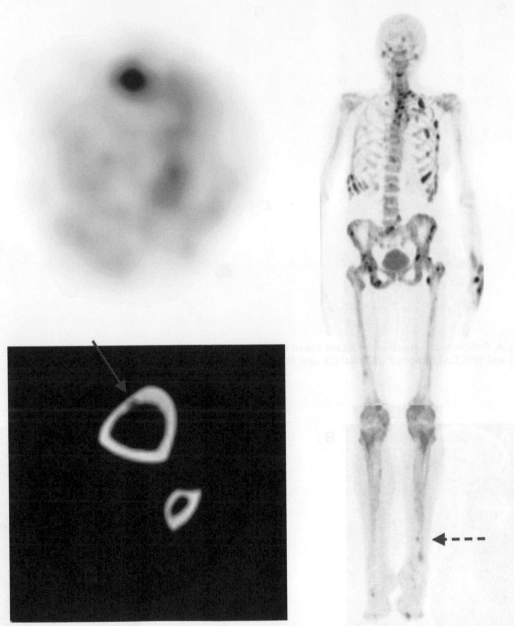

Fig. 6. Ability of NaF PET/CT to detect tiny lytic metastases. Focal uptake (*dotted arrow*) is seen in a 3-mm lytic lesion (*solid arrow*) in the left tibia in a patient with extensive metastatic breast cancer.

and oranges with oranges, not apples with oranges. Until such studies are performed, it can be argued that the advantages of NaF PET/CT, or at least part of them, are simply because they have been compared with planar BS with or without limited-FOV SPECT. It remains to be determined whether, and to what extent, the reported advantages of NaF PET are related to the tomographic acquisition, the higher spatial resolution and sensitivity of the

scanners, or whether there are biologic advantages of the NaF tracer (**Boxes 2** and **3**).

Review of published studies comparing BS and NaF PET demonstrate the limitations when only planar BS is performed and the added value of even single-FOV SPECT. One early study demonstrated the superiority of NaF-PET over planar Tc-MDP BS in patients with a wide variety of malignancies. NaF PET detected twofold more lesions

Box 1
Clinical indications for BS and/or NaF PET/CT

Benign bone disease

- Metabolic bone disease
- Osteomyelitis
- Sacroiliitis and ankylosing spondylitis[17]
- Arthritis
- Avascular necrosis
- Osteonecrosis[36]
- Paget disease[5]

Orthopedic applications

- Heterotopic ossification
- Painful prosthetic joints[37]
- Trauma and overuse injuries
- Bone grafts[38]

Malignant bone disease

- Primary bone malignancies[39]
- Metastatic bone disease[23,31,40–42]

Pediatric bone diseases

- Child abuse[43]
- Back pain[17,44]

Box 2
Advantages and limitations of BS

Advantages

- Tc-MDP
  - Wide availability
  - Generator produced
  - Longer physical half-life
- Lower radiation dosimetry
- Flow and blood pool studies (which often provide important clinical information)
- Favorable current cost effectiveness ratios

Limitations

- Inferior spatial resolution and sensitivity of gamma cameras
- Longer uptake time
- SPECT, and mainly WB SPECT is not routinely used
- CT to improve specificity is not routinely used

Box 3
Advantages and limitations of NaF PET/CT

Advantages

- Sensitive for lytic lesions
- Better resolution and sensitivity of imaging device
- Routine tomographic acquisition
- Routine use of CT improves specificity
- Shorter total examination time
- Accurate quantitation
- Superior pharmacokinetics

Limitations

- Cost
- Cyclotron produced
- Short tracer half-life for study logistics
- Higher radiation exposure
- Lack of flow and blood pool studies

than Tc-MDP, most notably in the spine and pelvis.[40] In a prospective study by the same group in patients with lung cancer, NaF PET detected 12 patients with metastatic bone disease, whereas planar Tc-MDP BS detected only 6 patients. Patients also underwent cervico-thoracic and thoraco-lumbar SPECT, which detected an additional 5 patients with metastatic bone disease, resulting therefore in only 1 false-negative BS study. Although the extent of metastatic disease was better assessed with NaF PET, this did not lead to any changes in patient management. The areas under the receiver operating characteristic (ROC) curves of NaF PET and Tc-MDP BS with SPECT were not statistically significantly different, leading the investigators to conclude that BS with limited-FOV SPECT is a practical and cost-effective examination.[41] In a larger study from the same group, including 103 patients with lung cancer, 33 patients had bone metastases. There were 13 false-negative planar Tc-MDP BS, 4 with Tc-MDP planar and SPECT of the entire vertebral column, and 2 with NaF PET. Clinical management changed in 7 patients following the additional acquisition of SPECT and in 8 with NaF PET.[42]

Even-Sapir and colleagues[23] performed a prospective study in 44 patients with prostate cancer that aimed to determine the optimal modality for diagnosis of bone metastases that included a subanalysis of a group of patients who underwent multi-FOV SPECT. Tc-MDP planar BS and NaF PET/CT were performed in all patients. Twenty of the 44 patients undergoing BS also had single-FOV SPECT and 24 had multi-FOV SPECT of the entire axial skeleton. The addition of multi-FOV SPECT improved the sensitivity of planar BS from 69% to 92% in the patient-based analysis, detecting 4 additional patients with bone metastases. On the lesion-based analysis, sensitivity also increased from 39% to 71% when multi-FOV SPECT was added to planar BS. Specificity in the patient-based analysis increased from 64% to 82% using planar and multi-FOV SPECT, respectively, and in the lesion-based analysis from 79% to 85%. NaF PET/CT sensitivity and specificity was 100%, using both patient-based and lesion-based analysis. Therefore, in this study, the sensitivity of 100% of NaF PET/CT in patients with prostate cancer was 8% higher than multi-FOV SPECT. Only 1 of 13 patients with bone metastases was not detected by multi-FOV SPECT, whereas the NaF study was positive.

Cost Effectiveness

Few cost-effectiveness analyses have been performed to date, all for NaF PET or PET/CT in metastatic disease. Hetzel and colleagues[42] compared NaF PET and BS (with and without SPECT) in patients with lung cancer. Cost analysis was based on direct costs (in Euros, €) of the procedures in German hospitals in 2002. At that time, the cost was 193.30 € for planar BS, 103.10 € for SPECT and 515.40 € for NaF PET. Three different cost-effectiveness strategies were analyzed. Strategy 1 consisted of BS with SPECT performed only in cases with inconclusive lesions in the vertebral column on planar scintigraphy. Strategy 2 consisted of BS and SPECT in all patients. Finally, strategy 3 consisted of NaF PET in all patients. A total of 87.4%, 96.1%, and 98.1% of patients were correctly diagnosed with bone metastases, for each strategy respectively. The average cost-effectiveness ratio in the first strategy was 252 €. The incremental cost-effectiveness ratio for strategy 2 was 1272 € owing to additional costs of 111 € per patient. The average cost per patient in strategy 3 was 526 €, resulting in an incremental cost-effectiveness ratio of 2861 € compared with strategy 1 and 10,016 € compared with strategy 2. Considering that there were 13 false-negative BS, 4 with BS and SPECT and 2 with NaF PET, this resulted in a change in management of 9 patients with SPECT and 11 with NaF PET when compared with planar BS alone. The investigators concluded that the routine performance of SPECT was the most cost-effective strategy in detecting bone metastases from lung cancer. Detection of bone metastases in 2 additional patients only with NaF PET cannot justify the twofold increase in costs using this diagnostic examination. The investigators further calculated that if the price of

NaF PET was to fall to 345 € or less, the incremental cost-effectiveness ratio of NaF PET would be less than 1272 € and would thus be preferable to the proposed strategy of routinely using BS with SPECT.

In a meta-analysis on the use of NaF PET and PET/CT for the assessment of metastatic bone disease, a cost-effectiveness analysis based on the overall accuracy of the 11 studies was performed. Using Current Procedural Terminology (CPT) rates for NaF PET or PET/CT, the average cost per study was $1000 to $1500 (US$) with a cost-effectiveness ratio of $1038 to $1558. For BS, including planar and SPECT, the average cost per study based on Centers for Medicaid and Medicaid Services rates for 2010 was $297. The average cost-effectiveness ratio was calculated at $404.[16] With shortage in supply of Tc-99m associated with rising costs, cost-effectiveness studies will need to be reconsidered and updated in the future. It should be mentioned, however, that the additional costs of subsequent treatments that may be altered or avoided owing to the superiority of NaF PET/CT were not analyzed in any study.

SUMMARY

Two of the most common agents used for bone imaging in nuclear medicine have been reviewed and compared. Tc-MDP with gamma cameras has long been used, and physician familiarity with this tracer is excellent. Cost-effectiveness studies and practicality of use are currently in favor of Tc-MDP. On the other hand, NaF is a very attractive tracer with many advantages and with the potential to become the gold standard in functional bone imaging. Certain limitations remain, with routine flow and blood pool imaging not yet feasible. There are only a few studies that have assessed the use of NaF in benign applications and more are needed, also comparing Tc-MDP BS and NaF PET/CT. Technological advantages with SPECT/CT and WB SPECT discussed previously may potentially allow Tc-MDP to compete with NaF PET/CT in the next decade. Ultimately, regardless of which tracer will be adopted for routine clinical use, we can rest assured that BS has a bright future.

REFERENCES

1. Blau M, Nagler W, Bender MA. Fluorine-18: a new isotope for bone scanning. J Nucl Med 1962;3: 332–4.
2. Collier D, Fogelman I, Rosenthall L, editors. Skeletal nuclear medicine. St Louis (MO): Mosby-Year Book; 1996. p. 4–5, 25.

3. Ben-Haim S, Israel O. Breast cancer: role of SPECT and PET in imaging bone metastases. Semin Nucl Med 2009;39(6):408–15.

4. Fogelman I. Skeletal uptake of disphosphonate: a review. Eur J Nucl Med Mol Imaging 1980;5:473–6.

5. Blake G, Park-Holohan S, Cook G, et al. Quantitative studies of bone with the use of 18F-fluoride and 99mTc-methylene disphosphonate. Semin Nucl Med 2001;31:28–49.

6. Wootton R, Dore C. The single-passage extraction of 18F in rabbit bone. Clin Phys Physiol Meas 1966;7: 333–43.

7. Czernin J, Satyamurthy N, Schiepers C. Molecular mechanisms of bone 18F-NaF deposition. J Nucl Med 2010;51:1826–9.

8. Grant FD, Fahey FH, Packard AB, et al. Skeletal PET with 18F-fluoride: applying new technology to an old tracer. J Nucl Med 2008;49:68–78.

9. Dworkin H, Moon N, Lessard R, et al. A study of the metabolism of fluorine-18 in dogs and its suitability for bone scanning. J Nucl Med 1966;7:510–20.

10. Donohoe K, Brown M, Collier B, et al. SNM procedure guideline for bone scintigraphy: Version 3.0, approved 6/20/2003. Available at: http://interactive.snm.org/docs/pg_ch34_0403.pdf. Accessed April 19, 2012.

11. Segall G, Delbeke D, Stabin M, et al. SNM practice guideline for sodium 18F-fluoride PET/CT bone scans 1.0. J Nucl Med 2010;51(11):1813–20.

12. Blau M, Ganatra R, Bender M. 18F-fluoride for bone imaging. Semin Nucl Med 1972;2:31–7.

13. Madsen M. Recent advances in SPECT imaging. J Nucl Med 2007;48:661–73.

14. Brenner W, Vernon C, Muzi M, et al. Comparison of different quantitative approaches to 18F-Fluoride PET scans. J Nucl Med 2004;45:1493–500.

15. Doot R, Muzi M, Peterson L, et al. Kinetic analysis of 18F-Fluoride PET images of breast cancer bone metastases. J Nucl Med 2010;51:521–7.

16. Tateishi U, Morita S, Taguri M, et al. A meta-analysis of 18F-Fluoride positron emission tomography for assessment of metastatic bone tumor. Ann Nucl Med 2010;24:523–31.

17. Lim R, Fahey F, Drubach L, et al. Early experience with fluorine-18 sodium fluoride bone PET in young patients with back pain. J Pediatr Orthop 2007;27: 277–82.

18. Xia T, Alessio A, De Man B, et al. Ultra-low dose CT attenuation correction for PET/CT. Phys Med Biol 2012;57:309–28.

19. Huang B, Wai-Ming Law M, Khong PL. Whole-body PET/CT scanning: estimation of radiation dose and cancer risk. Radiology 2009;251:166–74.

20. Douglas R, Cherry S. Small animal pre-clinical nuclear medicine instrumentation and methodology. Semin Nucl Med 2008;38:209–22.

21. Soret M, Bacharach SL, Buvat I. Partial-volume effect in PET tumor imaging. J Nucl Med 2007;48:932–45.

22. Eriksson L, Townsend D, Conti M, et al. Potentials for large axial field of view positron camera systems. IEEE Nuclear Science Symposium Conference Record. October, 2008. p. 1632–6.

23. Even-Sapir E, Metser U, Mishani E, et al. The detection of bone metastases in patients with high-risk prostate cancer: TC99m-MDP planar bone scintigraphy, single- and multi-field-of-view SPECT, F18-fluoride PET, and F18-fluoride PET/CT. J Nucl Med 2006;47:287–97.

24. Kwee T, Takahara T, Katahira K, et al. Whole-body MRI for detecting bone marrow metastases. PET Clin 2010;5:297–309.

25. Iagaru A, Mittra E, Yaghoubi S, et al. Novel strategy for a cocktail 18F-Fluoride and 18F-FDG PET/CT scan for evaluation of malignancy: results of the pilot-phase study. J Nucl Med 2009;50:501–5.

26. Lin F, Rao J, Mittra E, et al. Prospective comparison of combined 18F-FDG and 18F-NaF PET/CT vs. 18F-FDG PET/CT imaging for detection of malignancy. Eur J Nucl Med Mol Imaging 2012;39:262–70.

27. Niederkohr R. Technical feasibility vs. clinical utility: a question of "can we?" vs. "should we?" Eur J Nucl Med Mol Imaging 2012;39:260–1.

28. Matsunari I, Kanayama S, Yoneyama T, et al. Myocardial distribution of 18F-FDG and 99mTc-sestamibi on dual-isotope simultaneous acquisition SPET compared with PET. Eur J Nucl Med Mol Imaging 2002;29:1357–64.

29. Slart R, Bax J, de Boer J, et al. Comparison of 99mTc-sestamibi/18FDG DISA SPECT with PET for the detection of viability in patients with coronary artery disease and left ventricular dysfunction. Eur J Nucl Med Mol Imaging 2005;32:972–9.

30. Gnanasegaran G, Cook G, Adamson K, et al. Patterns, variants, artifacts, and pitfalls in conventional radionuclide bone imaging and SPECT/CT. Semin Nucl Med 2009;39:380–95.

31. Even-Sapir E, Metser U, Flusser G, et al. Assessment of malignant skeletal disease: initial experience with 18F-fluoride PET/CT and comparison between 18F-fluoride PET and 18F-fluroide PET/CT. J Nucl Med 2004;45:272–8.

32. Kawaguchi M, Tateishi U, Shizukuishi K, et al. 18F-fluoride uptake in bone metastasis: morphologic and metabolic analysis on integrated PET/CT. Ann Nucl Med 2010;24:241–7.

33. Beheshti M, Vali R, Waldenberger P, et al. Detection of bone metastases in patients with prostate cancer by 18F fluorocholine and 18F fluoride PET–CT: a comparative study. Eur J Nucl Med Mol Imaging 2008;35:1766–74.

34. Cook G, Parker C, Chua S, et al. 18F-fluoride PET: changes in uptake as a method to assess response in bone metastases from castrate-resistant prostate cancer patients treated with 223Ra-chloride (Alpharadin). EJNMMI Res 2011;1:4–9.

35. Ritt P, Vija H, Hornegger J, et al. Absolute quantification in SPECT. Eur J Nucl Med Mol Imaging 2011;38: S69–77.

36. Dasa V, Adbel-Nabi H, Anders M, et al. F-18 fluoride positron emission tomography of the hip for osteonecrosis. Clin Orthop Relat Res 2008;466:1081–6.

37. Sterner T, Pink R, Freudenberg L, et al. The role of [18F]fluoride positron emission tomography in the early detection of aseptic loosening of total knee arthroplasty. Int J Surg 2007;5:99–104.

38. Berding G, Burchert W, van den Hoff W, et al. Evaluation of the incorporation of bone grafts used in maxillofacial surgery with [18F]fluoride ion and dynamic positron emission tomography. Eur J Nucl Med Mol Imaging 1995;22:1133–40.

39. Brenner W, Bohuslavizki K, Eary J. PET imaging of osteosarcoma. J Nucl Med 2003;44:930–42.

40. Schirrmeister H, Guhlmann A, Elsner K, et al. Sensitivity in detecting osseous lesions depends on anatomic localization: planar bone scintigraphy versus 18F PET. J Nucl Med 1999;40:1623–9.

41. Schirrmeister H, Glatting G, Hetzel J, et al. Prospective evaluation of the clinical value of planar bone scans, SPECT, and 18F-Labeled NaF PET in newly diagnosed lung cancer. J Nucl Med 2001;42: 1800–4.

42. Hetzel M, Arslandemir C, Konig H, et al. F-18 NaF PET for detection of bone metastases in lung cancer: accuracy, cost-effectiveness, and impact on patient management. J Bone Miner Res 2003; 18:2206–14.

43. Drubach L, Johnston P, Newton A, et al. Skeletal trauma in child abuse: Detection with 18F-NaF PET. Radiology 2010;255:173–81.

44. Ovadia D, Metser U, Lievshitz G, et al. Back pain in adolescents: assessment with integrated 18F-fluoride positron emission tomography-computed tomography. J Pediatr Orthop 2007;27:277–82.

Value of ^{18}F NaF PET/CT in the Detection and Global Quantification of Cardiovascular Molecular Calcification as Part of the Atherosclerotic Process

Sandip Basu, MBBS (Hons), DRM, DNB, MNAMS[a],
Mohsen Beheshti, MD, FEBNM[b],
Abass Alavi, MD, PhD (Hon), DSc (Hon)[c],*

KEYWORDS

- ^{18}F NaF PET • Computed tomography • Cardiovascular molecular calcification • Atherosclerosis

KEY POINTS

- Detection and quantitative assessment of active cardiovascular molecular calcification by ^{18}F-labeled sodium fluoride (^{18}F NaF) positron emission tomography/computed tomography (PET/CT) is a novel concept of recent times used to investigate atherosclerotic lesion at the subclinical and active stage.
- The major advantage of ^{18}F NaF PET/CT is its ability to demonstrate active mineral deposition in the atherosclerotic plaque. Theoretically, this modality will be positive before overt calcification on CT when medical interventions will be most efficacious.
- Visual detection of calcification by ^{18}F NaF PET/CT is subject to the partial volume effect related to the very low degree of radiotracer uptake at the atherosclerotic sites.
- Calculation of global cardiovascular ^{18}F NaF uptake in the heart and arterial wall with automated software has been an innovative approach to circumvent the above shortcoming.
- Further research in this domain requires to be undertaken for clinical translation of this concept.

THE MAGNITUDE OF ATHEROSCLEROTIC DISEASE BURDEN AND ETIOPATHOGENETIC TARGETS IN FUNCTIONAL IMAGING

Atherosclerosis is generally considered as a chronic progressive inflammatory disease of medium-sized and large arteries and healing response to endothelial cell injury,[1] often presenting as clinical cardiovascular disease events. The main clinical manifestations of atherosclerosis are coronary artery disease, cerebrovascular disease, and peripheral arterial disease, which occur in 2 of 3 men

Conflicts of Interest: None Declared.
[a] Radiation Medicine Centre, Bhabha Atomic Research Centre, Tata Memorial Hospital Annexe, Jerbai Wadia Road, Parel, Mumbai 400012, Maharashtra, India; [b] Department of Nuclear Medicine and Endocrinology, PET-CT Center LINZ, St Vincent's Hospital, Seilerstaette 4, A-4010, Linz, Austria; [c] Division of Nuclear Medicine, Hospital of the University of Pennsylvania, University of Pennsylvania School of Medicine, 3400 Spruce Street, Philadelphia, PA 19104, USA
* Corresponding author.
E-mail address: abass.alavi@uphs.upenn.edu

PET Clin 7 (2012) 329–339
doi:10.1016/j.cpet.2012.04.006
1556-8598/12/$ – see front matter © 2012 Published by Elsevier Inc.

and 1 in 2 women after age 40 years.[2] This disease causes more morbidity and mortality in the Western world than any other disorder,[3] and almost 60% of deaths are due to cardiovascular disease.[4] The specific pathways contributing to endothelial injury or dysfunction in atherosclerosis are not completely understood; however, well-known risk factors such as hypertension, hypercholesterolemia, toxins from cigarette smoke, homocysteine, and hemodynamic factors play the main role in

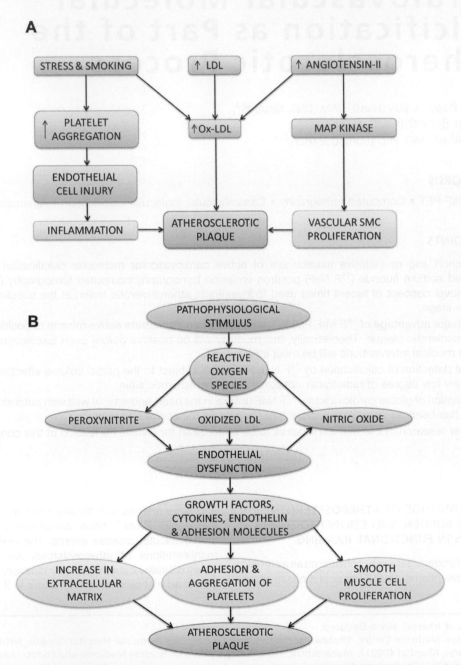

Fig. 1. (*A*) Schematic depicting the involvement of oxidized low-density lipoprotein (oxLDL), injury of endothelial cells, and proliferation of vascular smooth muscle cells (SMC) in the development of atherosclerotic plaque. MAP, mitogen-activated protein. (*B*) Schematic depicting the involvement of reactive oxygen species, endothelial dysfunction, growth factors, cytokines, and adhesion molecules in the genesis of atherosclerosis. LDL, low-density lipoprotein. (*Data from* Singh RB, Mengi SA, Xu YJ, et al. Pathogenesis of atherosclerosis: a multifactorial process. Exp Clin Cardiol 2002;7(1):40–53.)

this disease.[5] Nevertheless, there is substantial variation in the extent of atherosclerosis at every level of risk-factor exposure. This variation is mainly due to genetic susceptibility, duration of exposure, and other factors.[6] Hence, atherosclerosis may have a long asymptomatic phase, which can eventually lead to the occurrence of acute cardiovascular events such as myocardial infarction, unstable angina pectoris, and sudden cardiac death.[7] At present, screening of asymptomatic individuals and noninvasive measurements of subclinical atherosclerosis, including coronary artery calcification, intima-media thickness, and plaque of the carotid artery, is the subject of intensive research.[8]

Four distinct groups of targets have been attempted by investigators to explore the atheromatosis process[9–11] (**Fig. 1**): (1) atherosclerotic lesion components (targets include foam cells, lipoproteins, lipids, endothelin); (2) inflammation (targeting metabolic glucose activity, macrophages and monocytes, neutrophils, monocytes, and lymphocytes); (3) thrombosis (targeting platelets, activated platelets, fibrins, and so forth); and (4) apoptosis.

PATHOPHYSIOLOGICAL BASIS OF CORONARY CALCIFICATION: COMPARISON BETWEEN ATHEROSCLEROTIC VASCULAR CALCIFICATION AND SKELETAL CALCIFICATION

Certain facts about cardiovascular calcification need to be understood, which is important to further the proposed molecular approach of assessing atherosclerotic calcification; these are listed in **Box 1**. The mechanism and precise cause of calcification in areas of atherosclerotic plaque is not clearly understood at this point. The calcification in atherosclerotic plaque is calcium phosphate (hydroxyapatite), which is similar to that in bone. Thus, the theory behind the cardiovascular calcification has been proposed to be analogous to the biochemical mechanisms and substances implicated in normal skeletal calcification, with some distinct differences.

PEER-REVIEWED LITERATURE EVIDENCE ON DETECTING AND ASSESSING CARDIOVASCULAR MOLECULAR CALCIFICATION WITH ^{18}F NAF PET/CT

From the foregoing discussion, detecting and monitoring molecular calcification in atherosclerotic plaque appears an attractive target for functional imaging, and has been recently considered as an addition to the mentioned targets in **Fig. 1**. Thus, [18]F NaF PET/CT has been

---

> **Box 1**
> **Important facts and sequence of events involved in cardiovascular calcification**
>
> - Calcification is not observed in a normal vessel wall and hence, when present, is evidence of atherosclerosis.
> - The deposits of calcification are small, discrete, separate foci to start with, but active longitudinal growth of the calcific foci occurs with fusion of adjacent plaques following continuing wall injury caused by hemodynamic stress and other factors.
> - The extent and amount of vascular calcification tend to increase with age, but the process of calcification reflects atherosclerotic injury and only age plays no direct role toward its causation.
> - It is considered as a physiologic defense against active, progressive atherosclerotic disease.
> - The vascular calcification initiates with the formation of matrix vesicles derived primarily from degenerating smooth muscle cells (vis-a-vis in the skeletal system, they are derived from degenerating chondrocytes), which act as nucleators for the deposition of calcium salts in atherosclerotic plaques.
> - Calcification commonly takes place on the scaffolding of degenerated fibrous tissue, and begins with the exposure of hydroxyapatite present in the matrix vesicles to osteoid and to bone matrix proteins that are found in atherosclerotic plaques. Osteoid in atherosclerotic plaques are believed to originate from pericyte-like cells (vis-a-vis in the skeletal system, where they derive from osteoblasts).
> - The calcification process is potentially reversible with degeneration and resorption and the formation of a necrotic atheromatous core.
>
> *Data from* Refs.[12–17]

---

investigated for its potential to detect and image active cardiovascular calcification.[18–22]

In a retrospective study by Derlin and colleagues,[18] one of the early reports in this domain, the prevalence, location, and topographic relationship of [18]F NaF accumulation and vascular calcification in major arteries were evaluated. For this, the investigators examined 75 patients who had undergone whole-body [18]F NaF PET/CT for routine skeletal survey. Both visual and semiquantitative analysis was undertaken, and patient-specific and lesion-specific analyses were performed. On patient-specific analysis, [18]F NaF uptake was observed at 254 sites in 76%, and CT calcification was observed at 1930 sites in 84% of the 75 study patients. On a lesion-by-lesion analysis, colocalization of radiotracer accumulation and CT calcification was observed in 88% of the PET-positive lesions, whereas only 12% of all arterial CT calcification sites showed increased radiotracer uptake. The investigators also observed that a higher prevalence of [18]F NaF uptake visibility is related to a degree of calcification; however, they found no significant correlation between the intensity of radiotracer uptake (maximum standardized uptake value (SUV_{max})) and the calcification score.[18] It was inferred from these preliminary data that per patient the colocalization of [18]F NaF uptake and CT calcification was substantially higher than previously reported rates of less than 2% and 7% concordance of ^{18}F-labeled fluorodeoxyglucose (^{18}F-FDG) and CT calcification in other studies.

The same group[19] studied the correlation between [18]F NaF and arterial wall calcification in the common carotid arteries. Using semiquantitative SUV_{max} technique (by placing an individual region of interest [ROI] around the lesion on coregistered transaxial PET/CT images), they showed a significant correlation between [18]F NaF uptake and arterial wall calcification, as well as between the degree of radiotracer uptake (SUV_{max}) and both calcification score and calcified lesion thickness in the atherosclerotic plaque. [18]F NaF uptake in calcifying carotid plaque had a significant correlation with cardiovascular risk factors such as age, male sex, hypertension, hypercholesterolemia, and cumulative smoking exposure. Also noted was that the prevalence of carotid [18]F NaF accumulation increased with the number of risk factors.

In a recently published retrospective analysis,[20] fluoride uptake and calcification in major arteries (including coronary arteries) of 61 patients were analyzed by both visual assessment and SUV measurement. Fluoride uptake in vascular walls was observed in 361 sites of 54 (96%) patients, whereas CT calcification was observed in 317 sites of 49 (88%) patients. Significant correlation between the fluoride uptake and calcification was noted in most of the arterial walls. Fluoride uptake in coronary arteries was seen in 28 (46%) patients and coronary calcifications were observed in 34

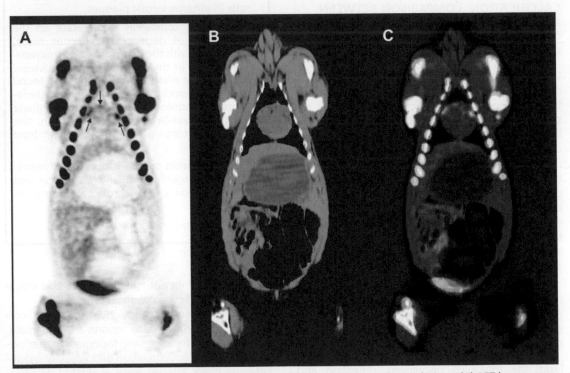

Fig. 2. Coronal [18]F NaF PET/CT images of a diabetic pig with known atherosclerotic lesions. (*A*) PET image generated 1 hour after the administration of [18]F NaF. Black arrows represent 3 sites of calcification either in the coronary arteries or in the soft tissues of the myocardium. (*B*) There is no or minimal evidence of calcification at these sites on the CT image. (*C*) Fused PET/CT image shows the location of cardiac calcification. (*From* Saboury B, Ziai P, Alavi A. Detection and quantification of molecular calcification by PET/computed tomography: a new paradigm in assessing atherosclerosis. PET Clin 2011;6(4):409–15; with permission.)

(56%) patients. There was evidence of significant correlation between history of cardiovascular events and presence of fluoride uptake in coronary arteries. The coronary fluoride uptake value in patients with cardiovascular events was significantly higher than in patients without cardiovascular events. The investigators concluded that ¹⁸F NaF PET/CT might be useful in the evaluation of the atherosclerotic process in major arteries, including coronary arteries. An increased fluoride uptake in coronary arteries may be associated with an increased cardiovascular risk.

The hypothesis of ¹⁸F NaF PET/CT in detecting molecular calcification of heart and major vessels of diabetic pigs was tested in the animal studies undertaken at the University of Pennsylvania (unpublished data). The animals were examined at different stages of the disease with both ¹⁸F-FDG and ¹⁸F NaF. The investigators reported the possibility of visualizing molecular calcification in the heart and lower lumbar aorta of diabetic pigs using ¹⁸F NaF before visualization of any visible calcification on the CT images (Figs. 2 and 3).

Global Cardiovascular Molecular Calcification Score: A Novel Approach to Assess Vascular Calcification

A novel approach was described by Beheshti and colleagues,[21] whereby the feasibility of ¹⁸F NaF PET/CT for the quantification of global molecular calcification of the heart and aorta was examined. The premise was that the modality could be used for calculating global calcification as a sensitive biomarker for detection of early molecular and cellular calcification in atherosclerotic plaques (Figs. 4–7). The concept was primarily based on the concept of global disease burden, which has been earlier used using ¹⁸F-FDG PET in a different scenario. In this study, 51 patients (34 women, 17 men) who had undergone ¹⁸F NaF PET/CT for assessment of a variety of malignancies were evaluated. Total slice volume and mean SUV in the defined ROIs on the left ventricle and different parts of aorta were used for quantitative assessment of molecular calcification score. The global calcification score was calculated by adding the entire set of measured molecular calcification scores in

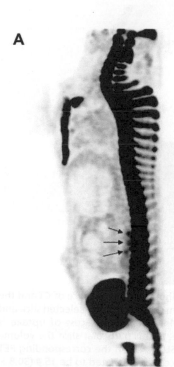
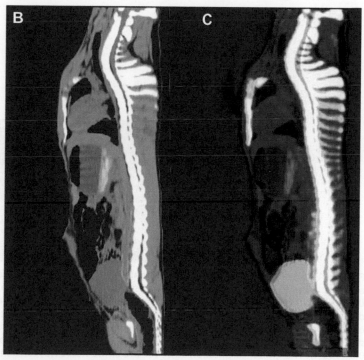

Fig. 3. The sagittal ¹⁸F PET image on the left (*A*), generated 1 hour after the administration of ¹⁸F NaF, reveals 3 sites of uptake in the lower lumbar aorta, which corresponds to sites of calcification on CT image (*B*), and their location is further confirmed by fusion images (*C*). In this animal model, this is the most common site for atherosclerosis and calcification, as noted in this particular study. There is no evidence of calcification in the descending or upper abdominal aorta either on PET or CT images. (*Reproduced from* Basu S, Hoilund-Carlsen PF, Alavi A. Assessing global cardiovascular molecular calcification with (18)F-fluoride PET/CT: will this become a clinical reality and a challenge to CT calcification scoring? Eur J Nucl Med Mol Imaging 2012;39(4):660–4; with permission.)

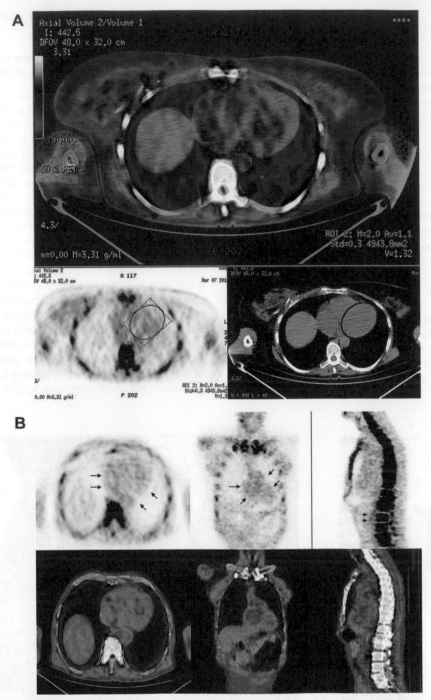

Fig. 4. (*A*) A typical region of interest (ROI) that was assigned to the cardiac silhouette on each slice of CT and the corresponding PET slice. The degree of ^{18}F NaF uptake is somewhat nonuniform throughout the selected slice and thus is of limited value for accurate assessment of related calcification. Moreover, the process of uptake is diffused and does not conform to the shape of the lumen in either ventricle. In this particular slice the volume of the selected ROI was 30.8 mL, and the mean standardized uptake value (SUV$_{mean}$) on the corresponding PET slice was 0.5. Therefore, the molecular calcification score for this particular slice was calculated to be 15.4 (30.8 × 0.5 = 15.4). The global calcification score for the entire heart was calculated by adding the individual slice values generated by this approach. (*B*) ^{18}F NaF PET/CT images of a 65 years old patient referring for the assessment of a cancerous disease. PET (*upper row*) and PET/CT fusion images (*lower row*) in transaxial (*left*), coronal (*mid*) and sagittal views (*right*): *black arrows* represent the sites of calcification either in the coronary arteries or in the soft tissues of the myocardium (*left and mid*) and in the abdominal aorta (*right*). (*Reprinted from* Li Y, Berenji GR, Shaba WF, et al. Association of vascular fluoride uptake with vascular calcification and coronary artery disease. Nucl Med Commun 2012;33(1):14–20; with permission.)

Cardiac Calcification

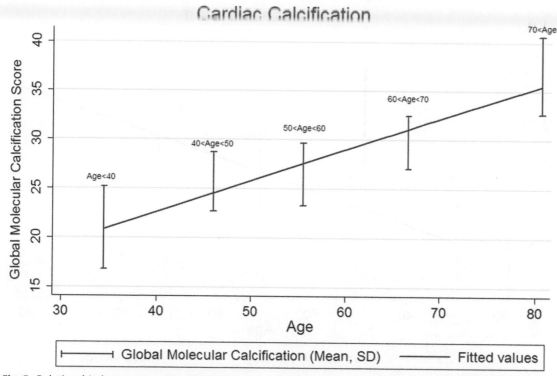

Fig. 5. Relationship between cardiac Global Molecular Calcification Score (GMCS), as measured by 18F NaF PET/CT and age. The GMCS data points (mean and standard deviation) reflect 18F NaF uptake in 5 different age groups. The fitted line shows a statistically significant increase in cardiac molecular calcification with age (Pearson correlation coefficient = 0.92; P = .003). (*Reprinted from* Li Y, Berenji GR, Shaba WF, et al. Association of vascular fluoride uptake with vascular calcification and coronary artery disease. Nucl Med Commun 2012;33(1):14–20; with permission.)

each ROI. The results of this study showed a significant correlation between measured global calcification score and patient's age. Based on these preliminary data, the investigators concluded that 18F NaF PET/CT may be a feasible modality for the assessment of molecular calcification especially in the early subclinical phases, during which no remarkable clinical and morphologic findings are evident.

This novel approach would require further validation by experimental and clinical studies, but opens up the possibility of a new armamentarium of functional imaging in the evaluation of this complex disease process.

Correlation of FDG PET, 18F NaF PET/CT Calcium Scoring: Implications and Advantages for Studying Combined Inflammation and Active Mineral Deposition in an Atherosclerotic Lesion by PET

Derlin and colleagues,[22] in a recently reported interesting study, compared and examined the inflammatory and calcification components by whole-body 18F-FDG PET, 18F NaF PET, and CT in the same oncologic patients. The macrophage activity was determined by 18F-FDG PET and ongoing mineral deposition was measured by 18F NaF PET in atherosclerotic plaque, and these findings were correlated with calcified plaque burden estimated by CT. Both qualitative and semiquantitative analyses were performed. The ROIs were drawn around the visually assessed lesions on coregistered transaxial PET/CT images manually.

18F NaF uptake was observed at 105 sites in 27 (60%), 18F-FDG uptake in 34 (75.6%), and CT calcifications in 34 (75.6%) of the 45 study patients. On a lesion-to-lesion analysis, 18F NaF uptake and CT depicted lesions colocalized in 77.1% of lesions whereas colocalization between 18F-FDG and CT calcification was observed in 14.5% of the lesions. Colocalization between 18F-FDG and 18F NaF lesions was observed in only 6.5% of lesions. The findings, the investigators concluded, suggest the distinctive nature of the pathogenetic processes and hence would indicate ongoing complex interactions between them

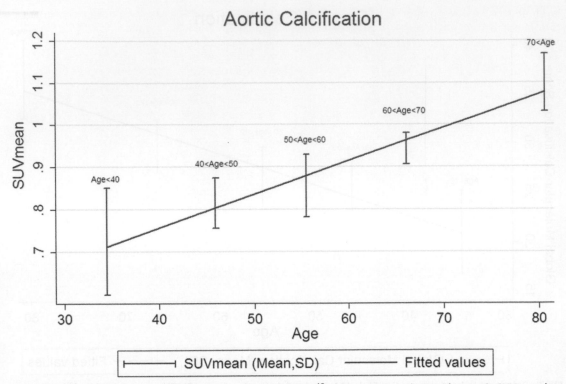

Fig. 6. Relationship between aortic SUV$_{mean}$, as measured by ^{18}F NaF PET/CT, and age. The aortic SUV$_{mean}$ data points (mean and standard deviation) reflect ^{18}F NaF uptake in 5 different age groups. The fitted line shows a statistically significant increase in aortic molecular calcification with age (Pearson correlation coefficient = 0.97; P = .004). (*Reprinted from* Li Y, Berenji GR, Shaba WF, et al. Association of vascular fluoride uptake with vascular calcification and coronary artery disease. Nucl Med Commun 2012;33(1):14–20; with permission.)

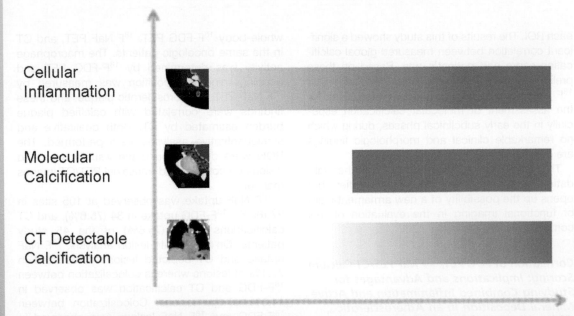

Fig. 7. Pathophysiological course of coronary calcification: a proposed schema. (*Reprinted from* Li Y, Berenji GR, Shaba WF, et al. Association of vascular fluoride uptake with vascular calcification and coronary artery disease. Nucl Med Commun 2012;33(1):14–20; with permission; and Diederichsen AC, Sand NP, Nørgaard B, et al. Discrepancy between coronary artery calcium score and HeartScore in middle-aged Danes: the DanRisk study. Eur J Cardiovasc Prev Rehabil 2011; with permission.)

in an atherosclerotic plaque. Also, the investigators hypothesized what may be perceived with the observed result, that ^{18}F NaF PET would depict active mineral deposition and provide functional information about the activity of the calcification process, whereas CT could only demonstrate the presence of mere calcification, which could be observed in active arterial calcification as well as passive mineral deposition.[22] **Table 1** reviews reported studies examining the role of ^{18}F NaF

PET/CT in assessing cardiovascular molecular calcification.

^{18}F NAF PET/CT VERSUS THE EXISTING CT CALCIFICATION SCORING: WHAT ARE THE ADVANTAGES?

Certain well-recognized limitations of CT calcification limit its reliability in adoption into routine practice:

Table 1
Reported studies examining role of ^{18}F NaF PET/CT in assessing cardiovascular molecular calcification

Authors,[Ref.] Year	No. of Patients	Global Quantification of Calcification	Setting	Important Observation/ Conclusion
Derlin et al,[18] 2010	75	No	Retrospective	Colocalization of ^{18}F NaF uptake and CT calcification was found to be substantially higher than previously reported rates of concordance of ^{18}F-FDG and CT calcification
Derlin et al,[19] 2011	94	No	Retrospective	^{18}F NaF uptake in calcifying carotid plaque had significant correlation with cardiovascular risk factors such as age, male sex, hypertension, hypercholesterolemia, and cumulative smoking exposure
Li et al,[20] 2012	61	No	Retrospective	Coronary fluoride uptake value in patients with cardiovascular events was significantly higher than in patients without cardiovascular events
Beheshti et al,[21] 2011	51	Yes	Retrospective	^{18}F NaF PET/CT may make it feasible to measure the regional and global calcification of the heart and major arteries; ^{18}F NaF uptake in the heart and aorta increased significantly with advancing age
Derlin et al,[22] 2011	45	No	Retrospective	^{18}F NaF uptake and CT depicted lesions colocalized in 77.1% of lesions while the colocalization between FDG and CT calcification was observed in 14.5% of the lesions. The colocalization between ^{18}F-FDG and ^{18}F NaF lesions was observed in only 6.5% of lesions

1. In an analysis studying coronary calcification versus luminal stenosis by atherosclerotic plaque, it was observed that 51% of all coronary segments with 50% to 80% stenosis, and 36% of segments with greater than 80% stenosis did not show calcification.[12] From these observations, one can infer that all plaques do not become calcified and absence of calcification does not exclude significant stenosis.[13]

2. The calcific deposits must be larger than 2 mm to be seen by electron-beam CT, and the reproducibility of the scans is relatively less.[16]

3. Inability to differentiate an actively growing, progressive plaque from an inactive, stable plaque on the basis of coronary calcification has been cited as a major shortcoming of CT calcification detection.

4. CT calcification score does not agree very well with respect to predicting future acute coronary events.[17]

Despite these shortcomings, it is to some extent accepted and proven that calcification plays a role in the pathogenesis of atherosclerotic plaque and the development of acute coronary disease, from the observation that virtually all acute coronary lesions are found to be associated with calcification. The major advantage of ^{18}F NaF PET/CT is that it would demonstrate active mineral deposition in the atherosclerotic plaque and thus would be able to address the last aforementioned shortcoming. However, the resolution-related shortcoming would persist even in this scenario, for which the global quantification would be a promising approach.

ASSESSING CARDIOVASCULAR MOLECULAR CALCIFICATION WITH ^{18}F NAF PET/CT: THE FUTURE

The assessment of "active ongoing" cardiovascular molecular calcification has recently generated significant interest among the functional imaging community. In a recently published editorial,[10] the authors had foreseen the potential areas where this could be useful. In this communication, the authors mentioned that one of the major limitations of CT coronary artery calcification (CAC) is the fact that it does not agree very well in asymptomatic subjects with clinical risk score algorithms such as the HeartScore,[23] and it is not infrequent to encounter CT CAC in healthy middle-aged individuals with a low HeartScore and, on the contrary, high-risk subjects with absent CAC. Hence arises the importance of ^{18}F NaF PET/CT in depicting

ongoing active molecular calcification in the plaque, which theoretically could precede the forecast of structural calcification detectable by CT. Atheromatosis is a complex process, and it can be presumed that both ^{18}F-FDG PET imaging indicating macrophage infiltration and ^{18}F NaF accumulation as a marker of molecular calcification would be pivotal to exploring and understanding the clinical course and the pathophysiology of the process. The global quantification of cardiovascular molecular calcification is an innovative approach in this domain that could address the shortcoming of the associated partial volume effect.[24]

REFERENCES

1. Libby P, Okamoto Y, Rocha VZ, et al. Inflammation in atherosclerosis: transition from theory to practice. Circ J 2010;74(2):213–20.

2. Rosamond W, Flegal K, Furie K, et al. Heart disease and stroke statistics—2008 update: a report from the American Heart Association Statistics Committee and Stroke Statistics Subcommittee. Circulation 2008;117(4):e25–146.

3. Roger VL, Go AS, Lloyd-Jones DM, et al. Heart disease and stroke statistics—2012 update: a report from the American Heart Association. Circulation 2012;125(1):e2–220.

4. Robinson JG, Fox KM, Bullano MF, et al. Atherosclerosis profile and incidence of cardiovascular events: a population-based survey. BMC Cardiovasc Disord 2009;9:46.

5. Libby P, Ridker PM, Hansson GK. Progress and challenges in translating the biology of atherosclerosis. Nature 2011;473(7347):317–25.

6. Greenland P, Abrams J, Aurigemma GP, et al. Prevention Conference V: Beyond secondary prevention: identifying the high-risk patient for primary prevention: noninvasive tests of atherosclerotic burden: writing Group III. Circulation 2000;101(1): E16–22.

7. Toth PP. Subclinical atherosclerosis: what it is, what it means and what we can do about it. Int J Clin Pract 2008;62(8):1246–54.

8. Greenland P, Alpert JS, Beller GA, et al. ACCF/AHA guideline for assessment of cardiovascular risk in asymptomatic adults: a report of the American College of Cardiology Foundation/American Heart Association Task Force on Practice Guidelines. Circulation 2010;122(25):e584–636.

9. Glaudemans AW, Slart RH, Bozzao A, et al. Molecular imaging in atherosclerosis. Eur J Nucl Med Mol Imaging 2010;37(12):2381–97.

10. Basu S, Hoilund-Carlsen PF, Alavi A. Assessing global cardiovascular molecular calcification with (18)F-fluoride PET/CT: will this become a clinical

reality and a challenge to CT calcification scoring? Eur J Nucl Med Mol Imaging 2012;00(4):000-4.

11. Singh RB, Mengi SA, Xu YJ, et al. Pathogenesis of atherosclerosis: a multifactorial process. Exp Clin Cardiol 2002;7(1):40–53.

12. Frink RJ. Calcification: a physiologic defence. In: Inflammatory atherosclerosis: characteristics of the injurious agent. Sacramento (CA): Heart Research Foundation; 2002. Chapter 5.

13. Wexler L, Brundage B, Crouse J, et al. Coronary artery calcification: pathophysiology, epidemiology, imaging methods, and clinical implications. A statement for health professionals from the American Heart Association. Writing Group. Circulation 1996; 94(5):1175–92.

14. Rumberger JA, Simons DB, Fitzpatrick LA, et al. Coronary artery calcium area by electron-beam computed tomography and coronary atherosclerotic plaque area. A histopathologic correlative study. Circulation 1995;92(8):2157–62.

15. Gutfinger DE, Leung CY, Hiro T, et al. In vitro atherosclerotic plaque and calcium quantitation by intravascular ultrasound and electron-beam computed tomography. Am Heart J 1996;131(5):899–906.

16. Devries S, Wolfkiel C, Shah V, et al. Reproducibility of the measurement of coronary calcium with ultrafast computed tomography. Am J Cardiol 1995; 75(14):973–5.

17. Detrano RC, Wong ND, Doherty TM, et al. Coronary calcium does not accurately predict near-term future coronary events in high-risk adults. Circulation 1999; 99(20):2633–8.

18. Derlin T, Richter U, Bannas P, et al. Feasibility of ^{18}F-sodium fluoride PET/CT for imaging of atherosclerotic plaque. J Nucl Med 2010;51(6):862–5.

19. Derlin T, Wisotzki C, Richter U, et al. In vivo imaging of mineral deposition in carotid plaque using ^{18}F-sodium fluoride PET/CT: correlation with atherogenic risk factors. J Nucl Med 2011;52(3): 362–8.

20. Li Y, Berenji GR, Shaba WF, et al. Association of vascular fluoride uptake with vascular calcification and coronary artery disease. Nucl Med Commun 2012;33(1):14–20.

21. Beheshti M, Saboury B, Mehta NN, et al. Detection and global quantification of cardiovascular molecular calcification by fluoro18-fluoride positron emission tomography/computed tomography–a novel concept. Hell J Nucl Med 2011;14(2):114–20.

22. Derlin T, Toth Z, Papp L, et al. Correlation of inflammation assessed by ^{18}F-FDG PET, active mineral deposition assessed by ^{18}F-fluoride PET, and vascular calcification in atherosclerotic plaque: a dual-tracer PET/CT study. J Nucl Med 2011;52(7): 1020–7.

23. Diederichsen AC, Sand NP, Nørgaard B, et al. Discrepancy between coronary artery calcium score and HeartScore in middle-aged Danes: the DanRisk study. Eur J Prev Cardiol 2012;19(3): 558–64.

24. Saboury B, Ziai P, Alavi A. Detection and quantification of molecular calcification by PET/computed tomography: a new paradigm in assessing atherosclerosis. PET Clin 2011;6(4):409–15.

Index

Note: Page numbers of article titles are in **boldface** type.

Moving?

**Make sure your subscription
moves with you!**

To notify us of your new address, find your Clinics Account
Number (located on your mailing label above your name),
and contact customer service at:

Email: journalscustomerservice-usa@elsevier.com

800-654-2452 (subscribers in the U.S. & Canada)
314-447-8871 (subscribers outside of the U.S. & Canada)

Fax number: 314-447-8029

**Elsevier Health Sciences Division
Subscription Customer Service
3251 Riverport Lane
Maryland Heights, MO 63043**

ELSEVIER

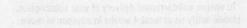

Printed and bound by CPI Group (UK) Ltd, Croydon, CR0 4YY

03/10/2024

01040358-0018